DIABETES

DIABETES

Caring for Your Emotions as well as Your Health

REVISED EDITION

JERRY EDELWICH, L.C.S.W.

ARCHIE BRODSKY

FOREWORD BY
RONALD A. ARKY, M.D.

A Merloyd Lawrence Book

PERSEUS BOOKS
Reading, Massachusetts

Material from "Another Point of View" by Joan Hoover is from B. A. Hamburg, L. F. Lipsett, G. E. Inoff, and A. L. Drash, eds., *Behavioral and Psychosocial Issues in Diabetes, Proceedings of the National Conference*, Washington, D.C.: U.S. Department of Health and Human Services (National Institute of Diabetes and Digestive and Kidney Diseases), 1979 (NIH Publication No. 80-1993).

Library of Congress Catalog Card Number: 98-87224

ISBN 0-7382-0021-2

Perseus Books is a member of the Perseus Books Group

Cover design by Suzanne Heiser
Set in 11-point Sabon by Vicki L. Hochstedler

123456789-DOH-0201009998
First printing, November 1998

Perseus Books are available for special discounts for bulk purchases in the U.S. by corporations, institutions, and other organizations. For more information, please contact the Special Markets Department at HarperCollins Publishers, 10 East 53rd Street, New York, NY 10022, or call 1-212-207-7528.

Find us on the World Wide Web at
http://www.aw.com/gb/

For Barbara
and in memory of Leon and Rose Brodsky

Contents

Contents

Foreword

In recent decades, the disease *diabetes mellitus* has come out of the closet, into the living room, and onto the television screens of the nation. What until the 1960s was kept as a deep family secret or, at most, mentioned to friends is now discussed openly on radio talk shows and in magazine articles and has even been the theme of a television situation comedy. This new candor about a common disease results from the efforts of a group of consumers – parents of insulin-dependent diabetic children who have been frustrated with the failure of the medical community to develop a "cure" for their youngsters. These parents mobilized and stimulated Congressional action, and through their lobbying efforts millions of dollars were allocated to support diabetes-related research. No permanent cure for diabetes now exists, yet these parents' efforts have led to an increase in our understanding of the disease and have helped to publicize it widely. In fact, the scientific knowledge about diabetes acquired in the last decade exceeds the total knowledge gained through all of previous history.

Advancements in immunology, molecular biology, and genetics have enhanced enormously the ability of physicians and other health professionals to understand the multiple factors that cause diabetes and to account for the great individual variability both in how the disease develops and in the occurrence of complications. The need to translate these scientific advancements into a language that has meaning and application for patients, their families, and friends is obvious. This book does just that. The authors neatly integrate the latest scientific facts about diabetes with the many mundane questions of everyday life that all persons with diabetes face.

So often, the physician, nurse, or other health professional responsible for the medical care of the individual with diabetes is too enmeshed in the biochemical or nutritional side of the disease and too busy to address everyday questions. The patient is left to struggle with how to acquire health insurance, select an appropriate physician, cope with the frictions and favoritisms that develop within families when diabetes is present, deal with questions of sexuality, pregnancy, and so on. This book is both a resource and a reference for these common issues. It provides guidelines not only for patients and family members, but for physicians, nurses, social workers, and other professionals.

Today we recognize that diabetes has many faces. In the past we considered the disease a monolithic disorder and made no efforts to separate those concerns unique to insulin-taking patients from those of patients who do not require insulin. Imagine the anxiety provoked in the middle-aged, obese patient who probably will never require insulin when she opens the manual given by her physician and sees pictures of syringes, needles, and individuals injecting themselves. The authors of this book distinguish between the two major forms of diabetes and spell out the unique problems presented by each, while recognizing that there are common areas of concern.

To understand is to care and to communicate. This theme, expressed so clearly and enthusiastically in the following pages, is the key to the care not only of diabetes but of all chronic disorders. A firm patient-physician relationship rests upon the mutual understanding and trust between the individual with diabetes and the doctor. This relationship also calls for open communication and an appreciation by all parties that the metabolic, psychological, and social variables that are characteristic of diabetes interrelate and

Foreword

influence each other. That people with diabetes like to be treated with respect, consideration, and compassion merely recalls that they do not differ from other human beings.

Too frequently, the diagnosis of diabetes spells gloom and depression not only for the patient but for family and friends. The period after diagnosis is difficult, and it is then that the common-sense, level-headed approach suggested in these pages is needed. For the reader with diabetes, this book is both an introduction and a guide. So many of the daily questions that you forget to ask your physician are answered in a frank manner. For the family member, there are explanations and helpful clues to account for the behavior or actions of a beloved one with diabetes. For the physician, there is an illuminating reminder that individuals with diabetes are in need of a certain brand of attention, compassion, and concern. The realistic view of diabetes that the authors present is an accurate compilation of the knowledge that medicine and the biological sciences have assembled about diabetes. The book also cites the many areas and problems about which we are still ignorant. But most important in these pages is the lesson that a rational and caring approach by and to patients with diabetes enhances the probability that they will lead successful and rewarding lives.

Ronald A. Arky, M.D.
Professor of Medicine
Harvard Medical School
Past President, American Diabetes Association

Acknowledgments

Some very special people have helped bring this book into being and keep it current. Harold Bursztajn strengthened our foundation not only by extending many professional courtesies, but also by sharing with us a perspective informed by discriminating thought and deeply meditated experience. Merloyd Lawrence, our editor, exercised judgment, skill, and patience in negotiating with us the long passage from conception to realization of both editions.

This revised edition would not have been possible without the major contributions of two esteemed colleagues. Barbara Puorro, research assistant for the New England Association of Reality Therapy, diligently searched both printed and online sources to pull together and make sense of the explosion of new information about diabetes during the past decade. We hope what she found will enrich the book as much for our readers as it has for us. Eric Lieben, M.D., went beyond the call of duty by not only updating, but also broadening and deepening the medical information in the book. His generous sharing of his time and expertise raised this aspect of the book to a higher plane of rigor and usefulness.

The revision also benefited enormously from Denise Bergman's sensitive conceptual and editorial input, Alessandra Priorelli's timely, respectful attention to referencing details, and Eden Stone's familiarity with what people with diabetes are thinking and feeling today and how they are expressing their concerns. Michael

Commons, Richard Feinbloom, Leonard Saxe, Maureen Sullivan, Janna Jacobs, and Anna Casey also contributed to the updating of the book.

Many caring individuals contributed in large and small ways to the first edition. These are people who have coped with diabetes in their own and others' lives – as patients and physicians, therapists and educators, family members and friends. They have talked with us, reacted to our ideas, made referrals and contacts, and generally inspired us. They are: Susan Barrows, Ellyn Benson, Deborah Bowers, Buzzy Chanowitz, Pam and Jeff Chowanec, Michael Commons, Patricia Downend, Loreen Fraser, Phyllis Harritt, Kathleen Havranek, Stephen Jacobs, Alyce Kaplan, Eric Kaplan, Andrea King, Peter Leveton, Kathleen Lomatoski, David Marrero, Daria Medwid, Patrice Miller, Polly Nodden, Sally Prentice, John A. Pryor, Sr., June Raposa, Stanley Sagov, Meredith Scammell, Jerry Spindel, Jackie and Hilda Sullivan, Bill Tucker, and Barbara Walsh.

Special thanks to Dr. Ronald Arky at Harvard Medical School, to Dr. Alan Jacobson and Linda Donaldson of the psychosocial unit at the Joslin Diabetes Center, and Cindy Hyatt and Berney Hull of the Diabetic Retinopathy Support Group at the Massachusetts Eye and Ear Infirmary.

For assistance with the revised edition we are pleased to thank Palmer & Dodge LLP of Boston and Kathleen Hickey of the New England ADA Technical Assistance Center for information about the Americans with Disabilities Act; Saundra Ketner, librarian at the Alexander Marble Library, Joslin Diabetes Center; the staff of The Learning Center at the Beth Israel Deaconess Medical Center in Boston; and, last but far from least, Vicki Hochstedler for a skillful and enjoyable collaboration over the proofs.

J. E.
A. B.

Introduction:
The Human Side of Diabetes

So diabetes has touched your life. Perhaps you were told – yesterday or fifty years ago – that you have diabetes. Maybe it is not you but a parent or a child, a brother or sister, a spouse, fiancé, or friend or colleague who must deal with the daily adjustments (physical and emotional) made necessary by this disease. Or you may be a health care professional, concerned about the difficult emotional questions connected with a chronic, ever-present illness. As Alan Jacobson, M.D., medical director of the famed Joslin Diabetes Center, puts it, you have become aware of "entering a new world, filled with challenges and constraints."

Having diabetes is like being dealt a bad hand in a game you never intended to play. Walking through the casino of life, so to speak, you see a table marked "Diabetes" and think, "I'll pass on that one, thanks. I don't really understand the game, but I know the odds aren't good." Suddenly you find yourself seated at the table – and down a pile of chips before you even get started. Even as you collect your wits, the dealer is laying down cards and picking up chips. You'd better learn the game while there's still time.

You didn't choose the game – or the stakes, which are higher than you would ever bet willingly. But diabetes isn't just a game of chance; there are plenty of choices you can make along the way, and important ones, too. There's skill as well as luck to this game.

We all have our long and short suits; there's no denying that. But you can learn to minimize your losses, win some big hands along the way, and find satisfaction in meeting the challenge. This book will show you how to play the game of diabetes with a winning spirit and a winning strategy – just as Jack Benny, Jackie Robinson, Mary Tyler Moore, and Billie Jean King have done. Your accomplishments may be in a different league from theirs, but there is no one who cannot transcend diabetes in his or her own way.

✻

No doubt you have seen lots of books about diabetes. How is this one different? It's different in two important ways.

First, until recently, books about diabetes have been written mainly for just 10 or 15 percent of the people who have this disease – the ones who need insulin injections to make up for the insulin their bodies can no longer produce. In fact, the great majority of people who have diabetes have not fully lost the capacity to produce insulin. They have what is called "type 2" diabetes, in which the body cannot make full use of the insulin produced by the pancreas. Unlike type 1 diabetes, in which the pancreas can no longer produce insulin and which strikes with seeming randomness, usually early in life, type 2 diabetes usually shows up after the age of thirty-five or forty and is associated with overweight and a sedentary life. Often it can be controlled by diet and exercise alone, although oral medications may also be needed. (Insulin is prescribed at times of unusual stress or when other treatments don't work.)

A booklet published by the American Diabetes Association to increase public awareness of type 2 diabetes was entitled *The "Other" Diabetes* – testimony to the lesser attention often given to this type of diabetes. Type 2, sometimes called "silent" or "closet" diabetes, is much less dramatic than type 1. You can work beside a person with type 2 and not notice it, since that person usually doesn't take insulin injections and doesn't experience the precarious, hour-by-hour, metabolic shifts that are the hallmark of type 1.

All you may see is that your co-worker is dieting and exercising to "lose weight." In addition, since type 2 tends to occur in middle age and since the complications of diabetes usually take at least fifteen years to appear, the complications of type 2 (such as heart disease) are likely to show up at a time in life when they might appear anyway from other causes.

Unfortunately, the same matter-of-factness that makes your co-worker look like any other overweight person may lead the person with type 2, as well as that person's physician and family, to overlook the true nature of the disease. Most undiagnosed cases of diabetes are type 2. This neglect is costly, because the complications of type 2 can be just as serious as those of type 1, and yet type 2 in many cases is considerably easier to treat.

While the number of people with type 1 is remaining fairly constant, the medical profession is rapidly becoming alerted to the type 2 diabetes "epidemic." As of 1997, approximately one in ten adults suffers from diabetes, and the great majority of these have type 2 disease.

Throughout the following chapters, therefore, we will attend carefully to the 85 to 90 percent of people with diabetes whose concerns have been slighted in most previous books. At the same time, we will not slight the visible minority who will need insulin for the rest of their lives. Instead, we will include case examples from *both* types of diabetes, to illustrate the emotional strains and tough decisions that arise in the life of everyone with diabetes.

Many of the problems which concern people with the two types of diabetes of course overlap. Moreover, as a result of advancing age, inadequate treatment, or other illnesses, some people with type 2 do eventually need insulin, whether temporarily or permanently. And even those who don't may fear that they will. This is one of the major emotional concerns mentioned by those with type 2. What is real for the 10 percent is a dread specter for the 90 percent. The fear, and the reality behind it, need to be brought out into the open.

The question of fear – and its relationship to reality – brings us to the second and more important difference between this and other books about diabetes. This is not just another medical guide giving detailed advice about diet, exercise, insulin injections, foot care, and so forth. There already are plenty of good books of that sort, like the readings suggested at the end of each chapter and at the end of the book.

In contrast, our goal is to take a deeper look at questions that typically are summed up in one chapter or less of the medically oriented handbooks, a chapter called "Emotional Factors" or "Psychosocial Issues." Questions like these: "How does it feel to be told you have diabetes?" "How does it feel to live with this disease year after year?" "How does diabetes affect your relationships with people close to you?" "How do those relationships affect the way you manage your diabetes?" "How does diabetes affect your job?"

In other words, this book is about the *experience* of diabetes. Other books tell you how to measure units of insulin in a syringe; this one lets you ask yourself whether you are embarrassed to bring friends into the house when your father is taking his "shot." How *do* you feel about that mean old mother-in-law who told her daughter "not to get mixed up with a diabetic"? It may be encouraging to read that by losing weight you can neutralize the effects of type 2 diabetes. But that raises quite another set of questions – when you consider that if you do get down to normal weight, after all these comfortably fat years, you may once again attract the attention of potential mates.

Facts about food exchanges, urine test readings, oral hypoglycemic medications, and telling the difference between an insulin reaction and a diabetic coma make up the *content* of diabetes care. Such details are vitally important. Equally important, however, is the *context* of diabetes care – the background of emotions, attitudes, and conscious and unconscious choices that have so much to do with whether you can cope effectively with this complex and demanding disease. Education about the "external" facts of diabetes is necessary. Yet often the people who are least successful in maintaining metabolic control are among the best informed factually, since they so frequently land back in the hospital for re-education! They don't make good use of their knowledge, because they haven't worked through their feelings, examined the basis of their attitudes, or considered the implications of their choices.

In contemporary lingo, it's a "heavy" thing to learn that you — or someone you love – has a disease that lasts a lifetime and requires constant attention. It brings up feelings of loss, fear, anger, guilt, frustration, helplessness, anxiety, depression, denial – a spectrum of intense emotional reactions. It sets up tensions in daily living and erects barriers between family members, friends, and co-workers, not to mention between the patient and that demigod/villain, the doctor. It takes more than well-intentioned homilies to get to know the feelings, the tensions, the barriers for what they are.

Words like "Don't panic" and "Don't let it get you down" are among the easiest said and hardest done. What good does it do to say, "Share your problems with your family; you can count on their support," when your brother is jealous of the extra attention you get because of your diabetes, or your spouse unconsciously fears the more attractive person you may become if you succeed in losing weight? How can you believe in a manual that tells you, "Always follow your doctor's recommendations," if your doctor doesn't explain the reasons for those recommendations? How can you have a constructive relationship with a doctor who seems inaccessible, inconsistent, or insensitive?

As the very existence of diabetes demonstrates, we don't live in an ideal world. Nature is complicated, and so are people. Some doctors and nurses really are uncommunicative, arrogant, or ill-informed. On the other hand, you may perceive your doctor in that light because blaming the doctor makes it a bit easier to bear the misfortune of having diabetes. Either way, the feelings and perceptions have to be dealt with before you can decide whether to find another doctor or listen to this one.

The silent anguish, the emotional conflicts, the tangled relationships with others – these constitute the "'inner game" of diabetes. You may recall a popular book called *The Inner Game of Tennis*.

It made the point that winning at tennis is not just a matter of strokes, but of attitudes – of mental as well as physical preparation. So it is with the serious "game" of diabetes. If you play the inner game well, you have a better chance to win the outer game, where the score is finally kept. As recent research makes clear, the better you understand – and master – your feelings, the better you can regulate your blood sugar (Cox and Gonder-Frederick, 1992).

It works the opposite way, too. Feelings of success are fed by actual success. One of the best things you can do to give yourself a sense of being in control, therefore, is to achieve some real mastery of blood sugar control and other signs of physical well-being. That's where the information in those medical manuals comes into play. But if the emotional context isn't properly attended to, the informational content can't do its job. It just sits there, lifeless, on the page. Besides, since your physical condition is never *completely* under your control, it is important to achieve another kind of emotional mastery – that of learning not to blame yourself for having "failed" every time your body doesn't reward you for following the rules.

Emotional mastery doesn't mean only resolving disruptive conflicts and irrational reactions that keep you from following the rules. Many people follow rules too uncritically (for example, people with type 2 diabetes who take unnecessary medications when diet and exercise would do the trick). Emotional strength and clarity of vision enable you to do what is best for yourself and others, whether that means going along with rules or questioning them. It is essential to think for yourself, ask questions, and be clear about what choices you are making and why.

Until recently, little attention has been given to this vitally important context of diabetes. As a result, a great many people who have diabetes or who work with diabetes have had nowhere to turn for help in coping with its emotional ramifications. Emotional and interpersonal issues are insufficiently addressed – often omitted entirely – in the training of physicians, nurses, and other health professionals. Trained counselors are not, as a rule, available in physicians' offices and other medical facilities to work with the patients and caregivers. However, more and more physicians are now acknowledging the importance of emotional support:

> The feelings of patients, family members, and physicians can become quite intense when problems occur or a therapeutic impasse is reached. Recognizing that intense emotions may arise can help prepare the physician to work closely with the patient during periods of emotional turmoil and disappointment. Hearing, tolerating, and acknowledging the patient's expression of painful feelings is a key aspect of establishing and maintaining rapport through such difficult periods (Jacobson, 1996b).

When the emotional side of diabetes is neglected, people suffer in silence, not knowing that others share their concerns. They may fail to use the information available to them and may work at cross-purposes with their families, their physicians, and (worse) their own deepest intentions. Life-and-death decisions are made by drift and default rather than by informed choice. We hope this book will contribute to reducing such unnecessary human losses.

✲

You hear people say, "'Oh, diabetes – that's nothing. You just take your insulin and you're okay." You know better. You know that type 1 diabetes is, in the words of Marlene Lees "like being expected to play the piano with one hand while juggling items with another hand, all while balancing with deftness and dexterity on a tightrope" (1983). That type 2 diabetes does not inspire such colorful imagery is part of its special poignancy, for it is an often lonely, day-in, day-out struggle to master personal habits that are most resistant to change. Either way, you know it's a tough act to live *with* diabetes without getting caught up in living *for* it.

You know how diabetes sets its sufferers apart while leaving them to all outward appearances "normal." You've probably even hesitated more than once before identifying yourself as diabetic, wondering each time whether "coming out" would bring support or a stigma. And that is only the beginning. A study covering ten years of national TV news broadcasts revealed that diabetes is not portrayed on the nightly news as a serious disease with sometimes fatal complications. What viewers learn is that people with diabetes need artificial sweeteners. But you don't have to watch TV to know that diabetes is a leading cause of blindness, kidney failure, sexual dysfunction, heart disease, and amputations – all told, the fourth leading cause of death in the United States.

An estimated sixteen million Americans have diabetes, eight million diagnosed and the rest undiagnosed. And the numbers in the United States and worldwide are growing. With better detection and treatment, people who have type 1 diabetes are living longer and are better able to have children (especially with recent advances in the management of pregnancy with diabetes). As for type 2, the dangerous combination of obesity, inactivity, and stress has created something of an epidemic of this more preventable form of diabetes in the United States and other countries undergoing economic development. (Native Americans have been especially hard hit, due to the combined effects of a high-carbohydrate diet, lack of exercise, alcoholism, inbreeding, and the stress of cultural disruption.) Both the rich and the poor are susceptible to diabetes, insofar as they tend to eat rich foods. Heightened stress seems to be an added risk factor among low-income families. Age is also a factor; the risk of developing diabetes increases in each decade of life between the ages of forty and seventy-five.

If current trends continue, a person born in the United States today and living seventy years has a one-in-five chance of developing diabetes. The economic cost of diabetes (including complications) is estimated at over $138 billion a year. Diabetes appears in the medical histories of an estimated 25 percent of American families and indirectly affects each family member. So, while the American Diabetes Association tries to find the eight million whose diabetes has gone undetected, let us also look to the often-ignored needs of those whose lives have already been touched by diabetes.

Introduction: The Human Side of Diabetes

The large and growing numbers that tell the public story of diabetes are important, but they don't portray the inner drama of one person suffering alone. Diabetes is experienced by individuals, both in the private realm of feeling and in families, friendships, working groups, and health care settings. These individuals represent a typical cross-section of human diversity – of wisdom and folly, strength and weakness, distinction and anonymity. Some of their names symbolize accomplishment in a wide range of endeavors: Giacomo Puccini, Thomas Edison, Paul Cézanne, Dizzy Gillespie, Ella Fitzgerald, Arthur Ashe, Waylon Jennings, Fiorello LaGuardia, Mary Tyler Moore, James Cagney, Ron Santo, Catfish Hunter, George Lucas, Andrew Lloyd Webber, Patti LaBelle, Jerry Garcia, Halle Berry – and, of course, Miss America, Nicole Johnson.

These famous names, together with the many anonymous heroes of the anecdotes in this book, refute all the old myths about diabetes. You've heard those myths: that people with diabetes can't hold down a job, can't participate in sports, can't travel, can't enjoy sex, can't bear children and shouldn't have them anyway, can't live a normal life span, can't. . . . These "can'ts" are like the "shoulds" and "oughts" and "musts" that psychologist Albert Ellis talks about – voices of negativism that keep telling us to live up (or down) to expectations. Ellis shows that we needn't be ruled by the "shoulds," "musts," and "can'ts." Instead, we can temper our sense of reality with a sense of possibility.

It isn't just the famous whose lives are instructive – and often inspiring. Groups (including those for families or helping professionals) are a way of getting to know some of those eight million friends you have out there. Groups, however, are not available in all localities. Managed care does not always reimburse the cost of psychosocial support. Also, not everyone has the time to go to meetings or feels comfortable doing so. Online groups are now available to help some people get in contact, but not everyone has access to the Internet or finds online contact satisfying. That's why we've based this book on interviews with people who, in one way or another, are living with diabetes. We hope that reading what they have to say will be like participating in a group experience.

Here you will meet all kinds of people: children and adults, type 1 and type 2, people with diabetes and their parents, lovers, counselors. People like these:

- A four-year-old who asks her parents, "Are we going back to the hospital to give back the diabetes they gave me the first time, or to get more diabetes?"

- An overweight man, newly diagnosed with type 2 diabetes, who reads all the diabetic diet books he can get his hands on, finds different recommendations in each, and exclaims, "What am I supposed to eat? Chicken three times a day?"

- A young couple, both diabetic, taking a long trip by train. The woman takes out her insulin and prepares to inject herself in full view of other passengers. "How can you do that?" her companion snaps, giving her a sharp look. "Aren't you ashamed?"

- A woman with type 2 diabetes who tells her counselor, "I'm so scared to lose weight because then I might find out that my husband isn't really impotent like he's been saying for the past ten years. And then I'd have to start asking some questions about how he's been shortchanging me"

Does any of these stories make you sit back and say, "Aha! That's the way it *really* is"? That *is* the way it is for a lot of normal human beings responding in normal human ways to an extraordinarily stressful situation. Some, through whatever combination of prudence and good fortune, have done very well. Others have complications far worse than you are likely ever to see; their realities are everyone's fears. They are all brought together in these pages to dramatize the chances and the choices, the spoken and unspoken feelings, the wise and foolish ways people cope. Some of their accounts will speak to you; others may not. But just as if you were hearing them in a group meeting, they will invite you to identify with the sadness, the anger, the poignancy, the humor (bitter as well as sweet) of life with diabetes.

In the chapters that follow, the word "you" will refer sometimes to a person with diabetes, sometimes to anyone who is affected by diabetes. If you yourself do not have diabetes, think of the "you" in the first sense as standing for your husband, wife, child, parent, friend, patient – whoever it is that you care about who has diabetes. Remember, you're still playing the game of diabetes; you're just playing a different "position" on the team. Your role as a loving family member or friend or caring professional is crucial in helping the person with diabetes win the game.

With diabetes, the inner game of emotions and relationships affects the outer game of good health in more ways than one. Exciting research is currently investigating how stress directly and indirectly influences the course of diabetes (Surwit and Schneider, 1993). We have a lot more to learn about the direct effects, but we already know what we need to know about the indirect ones. Emotional reactions affect our health by influencing the decisions we make and actions we take in coping with illness.

We don't have to await the outcomes of research to practice a commonsense approach to living with diabetes. Once we acknowledge fully both the medical realities (with all their uncertainty) and the equally real and important realm of feelings, we can deal with each realistically. How much immediate pleasure, personal comfort, or social belonging is to be sacrificed for blood sugar control or weight control? The answer to this question is not a matter of right or wrong, of being a "good diabetic" or a "cheater." It is a matter of recognizing the consequences of actions and assuming responsibility for choices.

As an earlier book cowritten by one of the authors, *Medical Choices, Medical Chances,* makes clear, good health is a matter of *probability,* not absolute certainty or uncertainty. We don't know for sure that maintaining good blood sugar control will prevent complications, but we know that it improves the odds. The odds, the probable consequences, are (in the words of psychologist William Glasser) the "givens" of the situation. Given the odds, we make personal choices. We're still taking chances (those can never be avoided), but the chances we take are affected by the choices we make – not only about insulin, diet, and exercise, but also about family, work, play, love, and sex.

Now there is growing evidence that the choices we make really do matter. The historic Diabetes Control and Complications Trial has demonstrated that keeping tight control of blood sugar can significantly reduce the risk of complications (DCCT Research Group, 1993). This massive study also showed that, with appropriate education and guidance, most people can change their living habits so as to achieve improved control (Lorenz et al., 1996). Signs of hope and empowerment are evident in other areas as well. The Americans with Disabilities Act gives people with diabetes a platform from which to fight job discrimination and negotiate reasonable accommodations in the workplace. On the other hand, the advent of managed care raises troubling questions concerning the adequacy of health-insurance coverage and one's right to choose one's treaters and treatments. Both in the area of job discrimination and in that of health benefits, diabetes activists are raising their voices in a collective act of self-assertion.

What's at stake in making the best possible choices? While nothing is certain, the approach and outlook dramatized in the chapters that follow can open doors to good health and a full life. The rewards within your reach are emotional strength and balance; clear thinking; effective action; and greater fulfillment in work and leisure, in friendship and love.

For Further Reading

American Diabetes Association. *American Diabetes Association Complete Guide to Diabetes: The Ultimate Home Diabetes Reference*. Alexandria, VA: American Diabetes Association, 1996a (paperback, 1997).

American Diabetes Association. *Diabetes in the Family* (rev. ed.). Alexandria, VA: American Diabetes Association, 1987.

Bursztajn, H.J., Feinbloom, R.I., Hamm, R.M., and Brodsky, A. *Medical Choices, Medical Chances: How Patients, Families, and Physicians Can Cope with Uncertainty.* New York: Routledge, 1990.

Ellis, A. and Harper, R.A. *A New Guide to Rational Living.* N. Hollywood, CA: Wilshire, 1975.

Glasser, W. *Reality Therapy.* New York: HarperCollins, 1989.

Jacobson, A.M. The psychological care of patients with insulin-dependent diabetes mellitus. *New England Journal of Medicine* 334 (1996b): 1249–1253.

National Diabetes Data Group. *Diabetes in America* (2nd ed.) (NIH Publication No. 95-1468). Bethesda, MD: National Institutes of Health, National Institute of Diabetes and Digestive and Kidney Diseases, 1995.

Raymond, M. *The Human Side of Diabetes: Beyond Doctors, Diets, and Drugs.* Chicago: Noble Press, 1992.

Rubin, R.R., Biermann, J., and Toohey, B. *Psyching Out Diabetes: A Positive Approach to Your Negative Emotions.* Los Angeles: Lowell House, 1992.

Simon, S.B., Howe, L.W., and Kirschenbaum, H. *Values Clarification: The Classic Guide to Discovering Your Truest Feelings, Beliefs, and Goals.* New York: Warner Books, 1995.

First Reactions

I

Have you thought how a family feels when one of its children is diagnosed diabetic? I think I can tell you. The cobalt blue that Picasso used in "The Tragedy" is a color almost impossible to mask or to cover – and that is the way it is with the feelings we are discussing. They never quite go away. Picture yourselves bounding into the scene of "The Tragedy" with your practice orange and syringe, your handy Clinitest kit, and exchange list. How would you expect to be received? (Hoover, 1979)

This quotation is from Joan Hoover, a prominent lay diabetes educator and parent of a diabetic child, speaking at a conference of health professionals. It captures the emotional impact of the initial diagnosis of diabetes – whether child or adult, type 1 or type 2. Here are some recollections of how it felt to hear the dreaded word "diabetes" applied to oneself or a family member. First, some reactions to the diagnosis of type 1 diabetes:

- Magazine illustrator, age twenty-eight (twenty-five at diagnosis): "I proceeded to freak out. I cried hysterically on the phone with the nurse and then left my office immediately. All I could think of was that I was going to die."

- Mother of four-year-old girl (age three at diagnosis): "I didn't think I'd make it through the first week. I'd look at this tiny kid with an IV in her and think, 'This isn't really happening. We'll go home and it'll all be over.'"

- Policewoman, age thirty-eight (five at diagnosis): "The doctor told me I had to take a needle to live. I felt like a prisoner."

- Student, age nineteen (sixteen at diagnosis): "I felt like my life from then on was just going to be a different life. I'd be sick and taking needles as long as I lived. I called my sister and told her I just couldn't take it."

- Rehabilitation counselor, age thirty-one (nine at diagnosis): "I was confused and crying on the way to the hospital; I had no idea what it was. My parents were calm on the surface, but underneath I sensed a subtle, harried frenzy."

Next, some examples of how it feels to be given the diagnosis of type 2 diabetes:

- Schoolteacher, age forty-four (forty at diagnosis): "I felt a sense of loss, a burning sensation, an 'Oh my God' feeling like when you lose your job or a good friend dies."

- Office clerk, age forty-seven (thirty-six at diagnosis): "When the doctor told me he thought I had diabetes, I said, 'Ha ha!' I didn't believe it. Six weeks later, when they stopped my glucose tolerance test in the middle and gave me some Uneeda biscuits and Tab – that brought it home to me. It was like a rite of passage."

- Social worker, age thirty-eight (twenty-three at diagnosis): "They found it out during a routine prenatal exam. They told me right on the spot; there was no prior suspicion. I just panicked."

- Homemaker, age forty-five (thirty-nine at diagnosis): "It meant not living, not doing the things I was used to – a total change of life."

- Truck driver, age forty-one (thirty-three at diagnosis): "The first thought that hit me was, 'How will this affect my family? Will I be able to go on supporting them?'"

As these remarks show, the emotional crisis brought on by the diagnosis of diabetes can be similarly intense for type 1 and type 2 diabetes. It is a major dislocation in life. At the same time, the second set of quotations is not as uniform in tone as the first. Type 2 diabetes is an adult disease of gradual onset. People often experience it in a less immediate, more reflective way than they do type 1 diabetes. When you are thirty-five or forty years old and are told you have a disease that, for the present, does not have dire symptoms or require drastic remedies, you may well have the time and emotional "space" to consider broader issues, such as the impact of the illness on your family.

The other side of this coin is the greater ease of denial with type 2 diabetes. With type 1, one typically does not say, "Ha! Ha!" and wait six weeks to take tests to confirm a physician's suspicion of diabetes. By then the signs and symptoms of serious illness are quite apparent – and scary. Sure, a child can be unaware of the permanence of diabetes, and an adolescent can deny the potential long-term consequences of neglecting this disease. But adults with type 2 can deny the very fact of having the disease, and this denial can lead to serious consequences.

Experiencing the Diagnosis: Type 1

Mary Ann was sixteen when she found herself, in her words, "falling apart." In three months she lost twenty-five pounds, leaving her "with only sixty-five left to go before I disappeared." It seemed she was always either drinking fluids or going to the bathroom.

She even wet her bed. That scared her – not to mention the embarrassment. It scared her even more when she started having trouble reading the blackboard in school. "All of a sudden the words would all run together," she recalls. "I'd put my head down on the desk, rub my eyes, and look up again, and it would be all right. Then it would happen again five minutes later." Neither she nor her family had any idea what was causing those symptoms.

Mary Ann was one of six children. Her father was immersed in work and kept a distance from family matters. Her mother did not take her to the doctor as soon as she might have, because she was preoccupied with another daughter who had just entered the hospital with mononucleosis. Her mother thought, in fact, that Mary Ann was sick from worrying about her sister. It was an aunt, frightened by Mary Ann's emaciated look and protruding eyes, who made an appointment with the family physician.

By the time she went to the doctor, Mary Ann's face was, by her own account, flushed and "sucked in." When she got home (it was in the afternoon) she fell asleep on her bed. A bit later her mother came in and woke her up. The doctor had called and said that Mary Ann had diabetes, with a blood sugar of 750. "Get her in here in five minutes and don't let her sleep," the doctor had told her mother. She had to go to the hospital immediately or she would go into a coma.

Mary Ann started to cry. She didn't know a thing about diabetes. Neither did her mother, whose only exposure to the disease had come through a relative who had contracted type 2 diabetes in her fifties. "I had no idea what they were going to do to me – just that I would have to take a needle," Mary Ann explains. "And I couldn't take thinking about it."

After Mary Ann was admitted, the doctor continued to speak mainly with her mother. As for Mary Ann, her head was a swirl of racing thoughts – that "my life from then on was just going to be a different life," that "I was going to be sick and taking needles as long as I lived," and the near-universal complaint, "Why did it have to be me?" At one point she called an older sister and told her she "couldn't take it," after which her sister came and spent a few nights with her in the hospital.

Mary Ann stayed in the hospital for two weeks, followed by two months of morning visits at home by a visiting nurse, who gave her insulin injections until she learned to administer her own. She quickly regained her lost weight, and her blurred vision cleared up. Looking back a few years later, she finds that life with diabetes only "half" resembles her dire and confused expectations:

> I thought I wouldn't be able to eat what I wanted to eat and do what I wanted to do. I thought I wouldn't be able to eat candy, chocolates, pastries, wedding cakes. That isn't true. I still eat those things, but I have to watch myself. I got used to those restrictions after the first couple of years. I thought I wouldn't be able to go out and have a good time with friends, and if having a good time means drinking, then that's true – I don't. It's funny – I never used to drink and eat a lot of desserts, but now that I have diabetes I feel like I want to do it all the time. And getting up late on Saturdays can be a problem, because there may not be any insulin in my body from the day before.

Beth was a commercial artist in her mid-twenties. Routine testing during treatment for an infection revealed sugar in her urine. The nurse asked her some questions. Was she often thirsty? Yes. Did she get tired a lot? Yes, but she was so busy it seemed normal to be tired. Did she feel a numbness in her fingers? Come to think of it, it seemed that she *had* slept on her hand several times lately. The nurse took a blood test and arranged to speak with her the next day.

The next day, a Friday, Beth was called out of a meeting at her office to take a phone call. It was the nurse, telling her that she had diabetes. Beth describes her reaction:

> I proceeded to freak out. I started crying hysterically right in my office. I really knew nothing about the disease. The nurse

told me I shouldn't worry; everything would be taken care of. The doctor would see me that afternoon; they'd call in a prescription to my local drug store; nurses would come to my home over the weekend to give me shots.

The nurse spoke in calm, sympathetic tones. Beth, however, found it impossible to be calm:

I understood the words she was saying, but I didn't understand how it all could be. She gave me a lot of data and definitions of terms that I must have asked for (I was reaching wildly for any information I could get!), but I wasn't taking it in.

After she got off the phone, Beth called a friend and said she wanted to come over. She then told a friendly co-worker what had happened and asked her to take over her work for the afternoon. With that she ran out of the office.

At her friend's house, Beth called a diabetes specialist recommended by her friend. The receptionist told her, "We usually put people in the hospital at the beginning. You need to be in a place where you can be monitored closely for a few days to stabilize your blood sugar." On hearing this, Beth "got hysterical all over again. All I could think of was that I was going to die." Beth sums up her feelings at the time:

I was in shock, the shock of disbelief. The previous evening I had discussed with friends the possibility that I had diabetes, and they said, "Oh, it's nothing; they just take pills now." These were intelligent, well-informed people telling me that "it's easily controlled now; it isn't the serious disease it once was." Then the next day I'm told I need treatment urgently. Nurses have to come to my home because it can't wait until after the weekend.

On the advice of the diabetologist, Beth went into the hospital that afternoon, accompanied by family and friends. Even with their support and with that of the physician, who came to see her even though it was Friday night, she remained "hysterical." She remembers vividly her first insulin shot, even though it was only 6 units:

> They told me it was no big deal, only a small dose, but I was terrified anyway. I've always been afraid of having shots; I don't know why. It's like watching films of drug addicts. The idea of it is repulsive to me.

Yet Beth had to learn to take care of herself if she was to get out of the hospital, and taking care of herself meant giving herself injections. She felt this dilemma as an emotional conflict:

> I knew my fear was irrational, in that the needles wouldn't really hurt me. But the first few times I just couldn't make myself do it; my hand just wouldn't go. My doctor had never seen anybody so hysterical. Finally I got him to give me a good dose of valium and learned to do it by sheer will power. After I gave myself that first shot I cried all day; it was a real trauma. From that point on I practiced and practiced, but it was a long time before it came easily.

Beth remained in a state of intense emotional turmoil for a week. "I couldn't believe this had happened to me," she says in retrospect. "It's so hard to believe it if you're feeling all right. I felt betrayed."

Experiencing the Diagnosis: Type 2

When Henry finally had a glucose tolerance test at the age of forty, he didn't feel any different from the way he had six months earlier, when a blood test had failed to confirm a physician's suspicion of diabetes. Indeed, he didn't feel any different from the way he had ten years earlier, when he had leveled off at thirty-five pounds overweight. So how long had he been diabetic? In retrospect, he felt that physicians had missed several opportunities to make a definitive diagnosis. For instance, six months before the actual diagnosis he had had a positive result on a routine urinalysis. He was instructed to return the next morning for a blood test, which came out negative. Only later did he question the fact that he had not been told to eat a big breakfast beforehand and that the blood test had not been a glucose tolerance test.

The tip-off that led to the diagnosis was Henry's mentioning that he took afternoon naps – something that he (like many people who do not have diabetes) had done most of his life. He was seeing another physician for treatment of high blood pressure, and this physician's careful workup turned up information (particularly about the naps) that led the physician to order a glucose tolerance test.

Henry's wife joined him the next morning when he returned for the test. While awaiting the results they both "gorged themselves on hamburger and a huge slice of cake." After lunch, the physician showed Henry that his test results conformed to the standard pattern of type 2 diabetes. Until that day Henry had barely considered the possibility that he had diabetes, since he had no diabetic relatives, no recognizable symptoms, and little indication that his physicians were concerned about this possibility.

Henry's wife remembers being "very upset" when they heard the diagnosis. Henry describes his own reaction in greater detail:

I felt a sense of loss, a burning sensation, an "Oh my God" feeling like when you lose your job or when a good friend dies. My subjective life expectancy changed. My father is almost seventy and weighs more than I do; he doesn't exercise and he has smoked for years. Yet he is in better health than I am. I always imagined that I resembled my father in his invulnerability to serious illnesses, as I did in other ways. Yet here I was at forty, first with high blood pressure and then with diabetes. The loss I felt was of my sense of immortality.

While Henry had strong feelings about his diagnosis, they were based on very scanty information. He knew little about the symptoms or the long-term complications of the disease. All he knew about was taking insulin, which did not apply to his case.

Henry was to learn a great deal, but not through the intense experience of immediate hospitalization. Rather, he learned through detailed discussions with his physician and extensive reading. Henry's story is on the surface less dramatic than Mary Ann's or Beth's, but it is one that is repeated all over the country many times a day, and represents a milestone for everyone who experiences it.

First Days

Our interviews reveal the depth of the emotional crisis brought on by the diagnosis of diabetes – not just by what is said, but by how it is said. One person might race through her story, event following event like a crashing waterfall. Another might intellectualize, while her precise recollection of early childhood scenes testifies to the deep impression these scenes must have made a quarter of a century ago. One interviewee goes through changes of voice in the telling – lower when he speaks of himself in the present, higher-pitched when he puts himself in the place of the child he once was. Another seems serenely above the battle – until he asks wistfully, "What usually happens to people who get type 2 in their forties?" or "Oh, so did that person die of it?"

Diabetes is deeply unsettling because it suddenly calls into question plans, expectations, habits, goals, one's image of one's life, and even life itself. If you have been through the personal and family crisis of newly diagnosed diabetes, then you probably will recognize some of the stressful, disruptive circumstances in which it occurs, as well as the major emotional issues that arise at this time.

How the News Is Presented

Health professionals cannot be expected to be trained psychotherapists. Moreover, with the pressures of managed care, a full appointment book, and a waiting line of patients, they have little time to offer psychological support. As a result, people often are given the diagnosis of diabetes without any emotional preparation. In an all-too-typical scenario, the patient comes in for a routine examination; blood tests are taken; the test results come back; the physician or nurse flatly announces, "You have diabetes," and discusses treatment.

Beth heard the diagnosis on the telephone in her office. In this way she was denied both privacy and the immediate physical presence of a supportive health professional. While most doctors who must give patients the diagnosis of a serious disease try to do so in person, the first diagnosis of diabetes is frequently given over the phone. One reason for this is the need for immediate treatment – itself hardly the most reassuring message. Nevertheless, the job of bearing the news is often delegated to insufficiently trained personnel.

Interestingly, Beth did not blame the nurse whose phone call upset her so much. She sensed that the nurse was sympathetic and that she recognized the devastating impact of the information, but didn't know how to handle the situation. It is a common plight for both patient and professional.

Too Much, Too Little, or Contradictory Information

The person – and family – with newly diagnosed diabetes is rarely able to receive detailed information calmly. If you have been in this position, you may recall yourself casting wildly about for any and all facts that might reduce the mystery and fear, even while you could barely retain the most elementary instructions. In this emotionally charged moment you may well have felt that health professionals were giving you too little information, thus leaving you up in the air about important questions, or too much information, thus weighing you down with issues you didn't need to face just then.

It is difficult for helping professionals to draw the right line here, since some individuals want to know right away about the likelihood of complications, for example, while others are better off waiting. The problem is compounded when you (or family members) speak with more than one physician or nurse and, not surprisingly, are told things (some of them, perhaps, second-hand) that sound contradictory. Often medical information is at odds with eagerly sought "folk wisdom," as when Beth's friends told her, "Oh, it's nothing; they just take pills now."

As a general rule, you and your family should not be burdened with too much information too soon. As Joan Hoover puts it, colorfully but wisely,

> These wonderful education programs planned for the first week the child is in the hospital might just as well be conducted in Chinese. Parents need only survival information at that time. (Hoover, 1979)

Misconceptions and Fantasies

What most people know about diabetes (unless a household member or close relative has had the disease) is folklore; it consists of a few concrete, vivid images that are at best incomplete and at worst inaccurate. Here are some examples from our interviews of what people thought diabetes meant at the time they (or their children) were first diagnosed:

> "You couldn't eat cinnamon rolls."

> "If you lived long enough, you definitely would go blind."

> "I wouldn't be able to eat candy and cake."

> "I would never be able to have children."

> "I couldn't put sugar on my cereal."

> "I thought if I married someone who didn't have diabetes, our children would have a fifty-fifty chance of getting it. If I married someone who did have it, our children would have it for sure."

> "I wouldn't live more than thirty years."

"It meant not doing the things that meant living for me, like cooking and baking."

These impressions are based on two major misconceptions. They assume that the diabetic diet is based on rigid rules and specific, absolute prohibitions, rather than the flexibility made possible by food exchanges. And they assume an inexorability about complications, hereditary transmission, and death that does not at all fit the facts, since these consequences are varied and largely unpredictable. The statement that you will go blind if you live long enough with diabetes might be true if people lived for 200 years. As for the last quote, cooking and baking in themselves never raised anyone's blood sugar. You can learn a great variety of new recipes that will not be out of bounds.

Children and adolescents sometimes visualize diabetes as either the loss of a body part or the addition of an extra part. Some teenagers imagine it to have been caused by their sexual fantasies – a version of the guilt reaction that, in different forms, affects adults as well as children, parents and spouses as well as those with diabetes. But the most poignant childhood fantasy about diabetes is the belief that it is temporary, that one can "get better" as one recovers from a cold or chicken pox. This is how one woman remembers giving up this misconception:

A few weeks after my diagnosis and initial hospitalization (at the age of six), I asked my mother for some Christmas candy. She told me in a kindly, gentle way that I still had diabetes and would always have it. My parents probably assumed I understood that already. But as far as I was concerned, if it hadn't killed me and if I was out of the hospital and felt okay, then I was cured! When my mother told me the truth I felt disappointed, helpless. My sense of loss was greater then than after the original diagnosis. It was like when someone you love isn't ever coming home again.

It is not only children who, in those first weeks of living with diabetes, harbor the wish that "if I got diabetes because I was 'bad,' maybe, if I'm 'good' from now on. . . ."

Reactions Based on Family History

Sometimes the problem is knowing too much rather than too little. On the one hand, a history of diabetes in the immediate family usually spares the newly diagnosed person and other family members from the more extreme fantasies mentioned earlier. If one of your parents has had diabetes, you are probably more realistic about food exchanges, insulin, and the compromises, concessions, and flexibilities of daily life than someone who has had no exposure to the disease.

On the other hand, you may also know more than you want to know about the long-term complications of diabetes. This is especially true for type 2, which has a higher rate of hereditary transmission than type 1 and is more likely to appear in successive generations of the same family. As one woman put it, "When I was diagnosed at the age of thirty-five, my first thought was of my mother. I couldn't help but reflect that she was diagnosed at the same age and has deteriorated ever since, despite having followed her diet strictly. It doesn't feel very good for me to see my mother going in for laser beam treatments for her eyes." If you have had a discouraging view of diabetes in previous generations of your family, bear in mind that, with better management and more precise methods of blood sugar control, the prospects for a person diagnosed today may be considerably better.

Yet a family history of diabetes can also have the opposite effect – that of making the disease seem more familiar, less frightening, and even (oddly enough) normal. Here is a remarkable account by a woman who was diagnosed twenty years earlier at the age of fifteen:

I was writing a report on diabetes for a high school class because my mother and two of my four brothers and sisters already had it. I went to the bathroom, tested my urine, and got a high positive reading. So my mother gave me a shot of her insulin, and I went to the hospital the next day. My mother was not upset, and I wasn't either. If anything, I was happy, because having diabetes made me more like my mother. My mother was a hard person to please, and maybe this was the way to do it. I started

*giving myself insulin shots right away without any difficulty. I
don't recall any big adjustment in my living habits. Diabetes just
seemed a part of living in that family.*

This is one of several atypical "first reactions" unearthed by our
interviews. A ten-year-old boy was pleased to find himself suddenly the center of attention in his family. He could be independent
when he needed to be (within weeks he was taking his own injections so that he could visit relatives overnight), but he was also
adept at using his diabetes as an excuse to avoid parental demands
and discipline. A girl in her early teens said to herself, "This is really neat. Now I get to learn to give shots." Finally, as a general rule,
first reactions are less severe in the elderly, for whom the diagnosis
of illness is not an unexpected occurrence.

Hospitalization

The immediate hospitalization that sometimes follows the diagnosis of diabetes, especially type 1, can be emotionally traumatic in
several ways. Having to go to the hospital right away creates a
sense of dire emergency, an acute beginning to a chronic illness.
For most children and adolescents and some young adults it is the
first time they have ever had to spend a night in the hospital.
Children face several hardships: unfamiliar surroundings, separation from parents, fear of the medical procedures that lie in wait.

If going to the hospital is a crisis, so is coming home. All of a
sudden the child who has been taken care of by experts becomes
the responsibility of the parents; the adult who has been a medical
patient must learn self-reliance in what is still an unfamiliar and
frightening situation. Complicating the hospital discharge is the
strong likelihood that insulin dosages will have to be adjusted in
the home environment.

Clearly, the hospital can be the right place to stabilize the condition of the acutely ill and to provide intensive testing and education. But learning to regulate your blood sugar in the hospital is
not the same as regulating it in the environment where you actually spend your life. Since leaving as well as entering the hospital

represents a dislocation, even a crisis, for the person newly diagnosed with diabetes, diabetes specialists increasingly recommend carrying out the initial treatment at home whenever feasible. Diabetes education proceeds more slowly and gradually at home, but it takes place in the context of "real life" where it will actually be applied.

Remission

After type 1 diabetes is diagnosed, there is sometimes a temporary return of insulin production by the pancreas. In about one-third of all cases a remission occurs within a few months. During this period, which lasts from weeks to months, insulin injections are not absolutely necessary. Nonetheless, the diabetes manuals will tell you to continue the insulin, even if it is only 24 units daily. There are several good reasons for making this recommendation. Stopping the insulin may encourage false hopes of a permanent remission. It is easier, both medically and psychologically, to increase the dose of insulin when remission ends than to resume it altogether. Finally, discontinuing insulin temporarily leads occasionally to an allergic reaction to the drug when it is resumed.

The manuals are right. Psychologically, though, their sound advice comes under the heading of "easier said than done." A woman in her twenties describes her reaction to this dilemma – and temptation:

> I didn't see any reason to subject myself to the injections for the sake of 2 units a day. My doctor went on and on about it – the symptoms would come back, I might develop an allergy, etc. I just said, "I don't care. I see an opportunity, and I'm going to take it." I stayed off insulin for four or five months. When I had to start again it was very traumatic – not physically, but emotionally. I didn't want to believe it. I asked myself, "Why is this happening to me?" – the same questions all over again. My doctor was right about that, but if it happened again I would still go off insulin for as long as I could.

This kind of testimony doesn't make the advice in the manuals any less valid. But it does illustrate why the manuals are incomplete. Medically sound *content* is not enough. People who have diabetes also must confront the powerful connotations that a procedure like insulin injection carries. The need to take daily injections in order to maintain a basic physiological balance can be a blow to one's identity, to one's sense of wholeness and autonomy. This inner meaning is what we mean when we speak of the emotional context of diabetes. It is not an excuse for disregarding medical necessities. But it must be acknowledged, respected, and incorporated into this personal decision.

Accepting the Reality of Type 2 Diabetes

Type 1 and type 2 diabetes require different kinds of emotional adjustment. Type 1 blows in like a hurricane, threatening to obliterate life as you have known it. Type 2 enters your life insidiously. There seems to be no real reason for changing your living habits. Indeed, you may have strong reasons *not* to make those serious changes that must be made. Type 2 makes denial (like that of the woman who said "Ha! Ha!" and put off being tested for six weeks) both easier and more tempting than does type 1.

Consider the circumstances in which type 2 diabetes appears. The disease may remain asymptomatic for years, both before and after it is diagnosed. By the time you have it (or know you have it), you are likely to be older and more set in your ways than the child or young adult diagnosed with type 1. Moreover, the very habits that you need to change are probably ones that contributed to causing the illness in the first place. This is not true for type 1. Type 1 does not strike mainly those people who crave sweets and have a phobia of needles. Some people adapt easily to its regimens and even enjoy regulating their blood sugar closely. Type 2, on the other hand, does strike primarily those who have overeaten and have been physically inactive to the point of making themselves ill. That may make it all the more difficult to change. Yet, by giving a person more reasons to change, it may bring about a miracle –

breaking deeply ingrained bad habits and bringing about a new, positive approach to one's health.

For Further Reading

Hamburg, B.A. and Inoff, G.E. Coping with predictable crises of diabetes. *Diabetes Care* 6 (1983): 409–416.

Hoover, J. Another point of view. In B.A. Hamburg, L.F. Lipsett, G.E. Inoff, and A.L. Drash (Eds.), *Behavioral and Psychosocial Issues in Diabetes, Proceedings of the National Conference.* Washington, D.C.: U.S. Department of Health and Human Services, 1979, pp. 25–32 (NIH Publication No. 80-1993).

Rubin, R.R. and Peyrot, M. Emotional responses to diagnosis. In B.J. Anderson and R.R. Rubin (Eds.), *Practical Psychology for Diabetes Clinicians.* Alexandria, VA: American Diabetes Association, 1996, pp. 155–162.

Tonnessen, D. *50 Essential Things to Do When the Doctor Says It's Diabetes.* Plume, 1996.

What Is Diabetes?

2

Most readers of this book already know the basic facts about diabetes, having learned them from physicians, from books, or perhaps from experience. If you are familiar with diabetes and how it is treated, you may choose to skip this chapter. If not, it will give you the background knowledge you need to understand the emotional and personal issues that follow. Further details can be found in the Glossary and in the many books and other resources listed at the back of the book.

Diabetes mellitus (DM) is the name given to a (diverse) group of metabolic diseases characterized by high blood sugar *(hyperglycemia)*. Diabetes is the most common endocrinologic (hormonal) disease in the United States, with about 5 percent of the population diagnosed with one form of it or another.

In the vast majority of cases, diabetes is a primary disease. That is, it is not known to be caused by any other disease. In some cases, however, what has been a mild, symptom-free case of diabetes may be "brought out" by some other condition.

Diabetes is caused by the body's inability to produce sufficient insulin or to use effectively the insulin supply it has. *Insulin* is a protein hormone which is produced by *beta cells* in the *pancreas,* a large gland situated behind the stomach, and from there secreted into the blood. There it has two major functions. One is to transfer *glucose* (a form of sugar into which most carbohydrates and some proteins are converted) from the blood to the body cells, where it is "burned" as energy. Insulin's other function is to convert excess glucose to *glycogen,* which is stored in the liver and muscles as an energy reserve. *(Alpha cells* in the pancreas produce another hormone called *glucagon,* which stimulates the conversion of stored glycogen back to glucose.)

When insulin is lacking or cannot be used properly, the body loses its ability to process glucose. As a result, glucose accumulates in the blood – a condition known as *hyperglycemia* (high blood sugar). Some of the excess is excreted through the kidneys into the urine; thus, the presence of sugar in the urine may be a sign (though an inexact one) of high blood sugar. Whereas a normal blood-glucose level ranges from about 70 to 130 milligrams per deciliter of blood, the glucose level in a person with diabetes may fluctuate from less than 50 (during an insulin reaction) to more than 500 (during a diabetic coma). A glucose level of more than 150 milligrams per deciliter signifies possible diabetes; the diagnosis, however, must be made by a physician.

Meanwhile, the body's cells cannot obtain sufficient fuel from glucose, nor have they a stored supply of glycogen to rely on. (The latter is used up very quickly in the absence of a continuing supply of glucose to the cells.) Therefore, the cells burn protein and fat for the energy they need. The burning of fat leads to the formation of highly acidic substances called *ketones.* The uncontrolled accumulation of ketones, or *ketoacidosis,* is a very dangerous condition which, if untreated, can lead to coma and death.

Types

There are two main types of diabetes. Type 1 used to be called "juvenile-onset" diabetes; type 2 "adult-onset" diabetes. But since classification by age was not always accurate, the two types were renamed "insulin-dependent" (IDDM) and "non-insulin-dependent" (NIDDM) diabetes. This classification, too, broke down because people with type 2 diabetes sometimes do need insulin injections. Therefore, in a move away from a classification system based on treatment, the American Diabetes Association's Expert Committee on the Diagnosis and Classification of Diabetes Mellitus recommended simply using the terms *type 1* and *type 2,* with Arabic rather than Roman numerals (Expert Committee, 1997). The two types stand for very different disease processes, yet the two can often coexist in the same person.

Type 1 diabetes occurs when the body's own immune system destroys the beta cells of the pancreas which create and secrete insulin. This disease most commonly begins in childhood and adolescence, but it can occur at any age. People with type 1 diabetes usually are not obese. They are prone to ketoacidosis and require insulin injections to make up for what they can no longer produce for themselves.

Type 2 diabetes results from insulin resistance; that is, the body cannot make efficient use of the insulin it produces. It is by far the more common of the two types, accounting for at least 90 percent of all cases of diabetes. The risk of this disease increases with age, obesity, and lack of exercise; indeed, people with type 2 typically are overweight. It often runs in families, even more so than type 1, but the genetics are complex and not well understood.

Since type 2 produces relative, not absolute insulin deficiency, most individuals with this form of diabetes do not need to be given insulin. Hyperglycemia develops slowly, without ketoacidosis, and thus about half of all cases remain undiagnosed. Unfortunately, these individuals can still develop long-term complications.

In addition to the two main types of diabetes, there is a special form of the disease that affects pregnant women. *Gestational diabetes* is any degree of glucose intolerance which begins or is first noted during pregnancy. It complicates approximately 4 percent of pregnancies and must be treated to reduce the risk of fetal and maternal complications. Therefore, it is recommended that all but low-risk pregnant women be given an oral glucose tolerance test at 24–28 weeks. Approximately half of all women with gestational diabetes will develop diabetes at some point in their lives.

Diagnosis

Diabetes can appear in the most obvious or the most subtle ways. The diagnosis is easily made when high blood sugar or the signs and symptoms associated with it are plainly observed. On the other hand, diagnosis becomes difficult when the blood sugar is marginally elevated and when no signs or symptoms are readily detected.

In 1997 the international expert committee sponsored by the American Diabetes Association (ADA) established new guidelines to clarify and assist in the diagnosis of diabetes (Expert Committee, 1997). The rationale for these changes was that diagnosing the disease at an earlier stage would make it possible to begin appropriate treatment earlier, resulting in improved outcomes.

In addition, the committee recognized two categories of impaired glucose metabolism in which blood sugar levels are above normal, but not high enough to meet the criteria for diabetes. These are called *impaired glucose tolerance* (IGT) and *impaired fasting glucose* (IFG). These "prediabetic" stages are considered risk factors for future diabetes and cardiovascular disease. By identifying people with these risk factors, physicians can observe their condition more closely and begin measures that may delay or prevent the onset of diabetes.

Causes

Although the causes of diabetes are not well understood, investigation in the case of type 1 has focused primarily on three areas: heredity, viral infections, and severe physical and emotional stress. It is believed that these causal influences act in combination with one another. For example, genetic factors may make some individuals especially susceptible to a virus that destroys the insulin-producing beta cells of the pancreas. Alternatively, there is growing evidence that type 1 diabetes occurs when the body's immune system mistakenly attacks the beta cells. According to one hypothesis, this may occur when a virus changes the beta cells in such a way as to bring them under attack by the immune system.

With type 2, heredity is even stronger. There is greater likelihood that a person with a type 2 diabetic parent will develop diabetes than will a person with a type 1 diabetic parent. There is also another set of causes not involved in type 1, namely, obesity and lack of exercise. Thus, a person's living habits have a lot to do with whether that person, if genetically susceptible, will develop type 2 diabetes.

Prevention

At the present time, type 1 diabetes is not believed to be preventable. It may turn out that a healthful diet, exercise, and/or avoidance of stress can help delay or even prevent onset in some vulnerable individuals, but such cause-and-effect relationships are still speculative.

With type 2, the picture is much brighter. Many of those who might be genetically susceptible avoid showing any sign of this disease simply by eating a balanced diet and exercising regularly, thereby staying physically fit and keeping their weight within normal limits. This is one case where the best treatment is also the best preventive, and prevention is the best form of treatment.

Currently, researchers are studying a number of possible ways of preventing diabetes. With type 1 diabetes, immunosuppressive medications directed against the immune system's destruction of the pancreas are being developed and tested. If this destructive immune response can be held back or stopped, the progression of type 1 diabetes may be slowed or even prevented (American Diabetes Association, 1998c).

With type 2 diabetes, a major focus of research is weight control – the extent to which maintaining ideal or near-ideal body weight (as opposed to either extreme) can reduce insulin resistance and thus delay the onset of diabetes and its complications (Ross et al., 1997). In addition, researchers are attempting to determine the benefit of heading off type 2 diabetes by treating it in the IGT or IFG stage. At these stages, insulin resistance is high, but so is insulin secretion. By treating people who are at this stage, physicians hope to give them a more normal metabolic environment. The oral medications *metformin* and *troglitazone*, which reduce insulin resistance, are among those currently under investigation.

Symptoms

The symptoms of diabetes vary from person to person. Among the typical symptoms of high blood sugar are the "3P's": *polyuria* (frequent urination), *polydipsia* (excessive thirst), and *polyphagia* (increased appetite). Both types of diabetes may show symptoms such as weakness, fatigue, malaise, weight changes, and blurred vision. However, these symptoms tend to come on much more abruptly in type 1 than in type 2 diabetes. Often the disease escalates into a diabetic coma before it is recognized and treated, with an equally dramatic restoration of metabolic balance when an appropriate dose of insulin is given.

The symptoms of type 2 develop much more slowly and may escape notice for years. Sometimes this form of diabetes is discovered only when a blood test is taken during a routine physical examination. In other cases, without any prior indications of diabetes, a person may come to the doctor with signs of a degenerative complication, such as peripheral neuropathy or retinopathy. Improvement in type 2 diabetes resulting from changes in diet and exercise is likewise gradual and cumulative.

Complications

Diabetes has both acute (or immediate) and long-term complications.

Acute Complications

The acute complications of diabetes are immediate effects of abnormal blood-sugar levels. Low blood sugar can affect either type 1 or type 2, often as a result of overly aggressive treatment. High blood sugar results in dehydration as well as in two special complications: *ketoacidosis*, usually in type 1, and *hypersmolar coma* in type 2.

Hypoglycemia. Low blood sugar is a hazard of either form of diabetes. It is often a complication of therapy (i.e., overtreatment with insulin, altered eating habits, or increased exercise). One form of hypoglycemia is referred to as an "insulin reaction." It occurs, for example, when a person exercises strenuously and/or waits too long before eating.

Symptoms of hypoglycemia fall into two main categories: (1) those caused by excessive secretion of adrenalin (sweating, tremor, anxiety, hunger, fast heart rate); and (2) those resulting from altered brain function (dizziness, headache, blurred vision, confusion, abnormal behavior, loss of consciousness, seizure). The brain is affected because it cannot easily metabolize fats as an alternative to glucose as a source of energy, as other body tissues can do.

If recognized in time, an insulin reaction can be stopped by eating or drinking something sweet (such as orange juice, soft drinks, candy, or sugar cubes). If it is not treated, brain damage or death may occur, but only after prolonged unconsciousness. The primary danger in an insulin reaction lies in the improper treatment that results when this condition is mistaken for diabetic coma or drunkenness.

Ketoacidosis. Ketoacidosis, a complication of type 1 diabetes, results from insulin deficiency. It is characterized by elevated blood sugar and the formation of ketones from the oxidation of free fatty acids. It is an emergency that requires hospitalization.

The symptoms of ketoacidosis include the following:

- Weakness and fatigue

- Increased thirst

- Increased urination

- Dry skin and mucous membranes

- Blood sugar over 300 mg/dl, but not usually much higher

- Fruity breath

- Large amounts of ketones in urine

- Heavy, labored breathing

- Frequent abdominal pain

- Nausea and vomiting

- Altered mental status

Hypersmolar coma. In hypersmolar coma, usually a complication of type 2 diabetes, very high blood sugars are associated with severe dehydration and altered mental status. Because of the absence of ketone formation, some symptoms of ketoacidosis – such as nausea, vomiting, and air hunger – are absent here. Hypersmolar coma is an emergency that must be treated in the hospital.

Long-Term Complications

It is increasingly clear that the long-term complications of diabetes result in great part from the cumulative effects of high blood sugar. These complications develop, on average, 15–20 years after the first signs of diabetes. However, some people never develop these complications, while others develop them quite a bit earlier.

Atherosclerosis (a buildup of fatty deposits in the arteries) develops earlier and more extensively in people with diabetes. Contributing factors such as high blood pressure, cholesterol, and smoking further accelerate its development. The result is an increased risk of coronary artery disease, stroke, and *peripheral vascular disease* in the legs and feet, sometimes leading to *gangrene* (tissue death) and amputation.

The heart is affected either secondarily via atherosclerosis of its coronary arteries, or directly via the development of cardiomyopathy, in which the heart muscle is weakened. Hypertension accelerates this process.

The brain is affected secondarily by atherosclerosis of its cerebral circulation, which may lead to a stroke. Not only do strokes occur more commonly in people with diabetes, but the damage caused is greater, on average, than in other stroke victims.

What Is Diabetes?

Retinopathy caused by diabetes is the leading cause of blindness in the United States. There are two types of retinal damage. *Background retinopathy*, which affects the capillaries (tiny blood vessels) that nourish the retina, usually does not cause visual problems of any consequence. A small percentage of people with diabetes develop *proliferative retinopathy*, in which new blood vessels grow in the retina and leak blood into the vitreous cavity (the jelly that fills the eyeball). Proliferative retinopathy can cause temporary or permanent vision loss.

Diabetic nephropathy, or renal (kidney) disease, is the leading cause of death in diabetes. About half of end-stage renal disease in the United States is due to diabetes. This complication may progress silently for 10–15 years before the kidneys begin to leak microalbumin into the urine, which is its first measurable sign. Strict blood-sugar control can slow the progression of diabetic nephropathy. In addition, hypertension must be meticulously controlled, as it increases the risk of kidney failure.

Diabetic neuropathy (disease of the nerves) can affect any part of the nervous system except the brain. It rarely causes death, but is a significant cause of serious illness and disability. Specific complications that come under this heading include loss of sensation in the hands and feet (causing an inability to react to injury, pressure, heat, or cold), intense nocturnal pain, muscular weakness, impaired functioning of the bladder or intestines, paralysis of the eye muscles (causing double vision), and skin and circulatory disorders. Some of these conditions are intermittent and may disappear with improved metabolic control or simply with the passage of time, but specific treatments remain elusive. For many men, the most devastating form of diabetic neuropathy is sexual impotence.

Diabetic foot ulcers occur because of poor circulation and neuropathy. Proper foot care is essential for anyone with diabetes.

Treatment

Treatment of both types 1 and 2 diabetes includes an American Diabetes Association (ADA) diet, exercise, and modification of other risk factors for atherosclerosis (such as hypertension, cigarette smoking, and cholesterol level). When necessary, several types of oral medications or insulin in several forms may be used. Hospitalization is no longer required for most people newly diagnosed with diabetes.

Treatment for type 1 diabetes consists of one or more daily injections of insulin together with a carefully regulated diet and exercise. Insulin must be injected because it is a protein hormone that would be broken down by the body's digestive processes if it were taken orally. Instead of taking injections, some individuals now wear a pump that delivers a continuous flow of insulin (see Chapter 11).

A constant balance must be maintained among food and insulin intake and energy expenditure. This balance requires frequent small adjustments such as eating extra snacks during periods of strenuous exercise. Such adjustments, together with the setting of optimal insulin dosages, can now be accomplished with greater precision with the help of home blood-glucose monitoring. This procedure involves dipping a test tape into blood drawn from the finger and noting the change in the color of the tape.

Type 2 diabetes normally does not require insulin injections. Often, a balanced, caloric-restricted diet and aerobic exercise (if carried out so as to achieve weight reduction and physical fitness) improve the body's utilization of insulin so dramatically that normal glucose metabolism is restored. If diet and exercise alone are insufficient, oral hypoglycemic medications are used. Insulin is reserved for those cases where all other treatments are ineffective or for occasional crises such as acute illness (other than diabetes) or surgery.

Although the development of complications is not fully predictable, there is now clear evidence that tight blood-sugar control gives the best chance of preventing, delaying, or minimizing complications. The Diabetes Control and Complications Trial (DCCT), a landmark study whose main findings were published in 1993, conclusively demonstrated that controlling blood sugars to near-normal levels is a major factor in limiting the development or progression of diabetic vascular and neurologic disease in type 1 diabetes (DCCT Research Group, 1993). Specifically, patients domly assigned to intensive therapy (a regimen of tight blood-sug control) developed less (or less severe) diabetic eye, kidney, and nerve disease than those assigned to conventional therapy. The better the control of blood sugar, the greater the protection against organ damage. Although heart disease rates were harder to measure since the patients in the study were relatively young, there were indications of a reduced risk of both major cardiac disease and peripheral vascular complications. The most significant side effect of maintaining tight control was hypoglycemia. But the benefits decisively outweighed the risks (American Diabetes Association, 1998b). Another encouraging finding was that, under carefully regulated treatment conditions, rigorous treatment of diabetes did not reduce the quality of people's lives (DCCT Research Group, 1996). Although the DCCT was limited to type 1 diabetes, its findings and those of smaller, ongoing studies of type 2 diabetes suggest that tight blood-sugar control promises to reduce the development and progression of the long-term complications of this form of diabetes as well (Colwell, 1994; Lebovitz, 1994; Pollet and El-Kebbi, 1994).

Other precautions, such as foot care, enhance these favorable prospects. Finally, a well-balanced diet and regular exercise promote good health in many ways, some of which are directly or indirectly related to diabetes. There is thus ample incentive to practice responsible self-care and obtain high-quality medical care. For, as the rest of this book will show, people with diabetes can live long, happy, productive lives.

For Further Reading

American Diabetes Association. *American Diabetes Association Complete Guide to Diabetes: The Ultimate Home Diabetes Reference.* Alexandria, VA: American Diabetes Association, 1996a (paperback, 1997).

Beaser, R.S. with Hill, J.V.C. *The Joslin Guide to Diabetes: A Program for Managing Your Treatment.* New York: Fireside, 1995.

Nathan, D.M. with Lauerman, J.F. *Diabetes: The Most Comprehensive, Up-to-Date Information Available to Help You Understand Your Condition, Make the Right Treatment Choices, and Cope Effectively (A Massachusetts General Hospital Book).* New York: Times Books, 1997.

Prashker, B.A., and Subak-Sharpe, G.J. (Eds.) *The Columbia University College of Physicians and Surgeons Complete Home Medical Guide* (3rd ed.). New York: Crown, 1995.

Saudek, C.D., Rubin, R.R., and Shump, C.S. *The Johns Hopkins Guide to Diabetes: For Today and Tomorrow (Johns Hopkins Health Book).* Baltimore: Johns Hopkins University Press, 1997.

Shared Concerns

3

Certain emotional concerns are shared by virtually everyone who has diabetes. Some have to do with things that are pretty certain (the troublesome routines and sacrifices involved in diet and in taking insulin). But the most powerful emotions swirl around uncertain possibilities (social isolation, the inability to work or to have a normal family life, physical disability, and death). They represent concerns about the future – a future made more uncertain by the questions raised by diabetes.

Questions on Everyone's Mind

Perhaps you have already heard yourself or someone else ask questions like these:

"Do I have to think about diabetes every minute of the day?"

It is often said that diabetes is a twenty-four-hour-a-day job, one that leaves a person susceptible to "burnout" (Polonsky, 1996). Here is one man's way of saying it:

Diabetes dictates pretty much your entire life. Unless you've lived through it, you can't really appreciate the omnipresence of the disease for the diabetic person and spouse during all their waking hours.

This is more obviously true of type 1 diabetes, where "metabolic chaos is always just around the corner and, to prevent it, subtle and constant shifts in equilibrium must be taken care of every day" (Monagan, 1982). But type 2 diabetes is also a day-to-day job, though in a different way. It does not involve hourly metabolic adjustments or the ever-present peril of an insulin reaction, but it does require a constant commitment to live differently from before – to exercise, to refrain from eating and drinking all those old familiar things, to learn a new set of habits. That, too, takes concentration.

When you have diabetes you run the risk of appearing overly self-preoccupied. As Joan Hoover has noted:

If your EVERY DAY *includes:*

- *I need my shot,*

- *I must test my urine,*

- *I need to eat, right now!,*

- *I have to have just the right food in just the right quantity,*

- *I need exercise,*

- *I feel shaky and need help,*

before long you become a very self-centered, me-first kind of person (Hoover, 1979).

People react to this regime in different ways. Some, surprisingly enough, thrive on it emotionally. People, like engineers and accountants who excel at precise detail work, may adapt well to routines that others find a crushing burden. They may deal with their grief and fear by relishing the intricacies of insulin dosage and administration. Children previously diagnosed as hyperkinetic and adults who have been unemployed may find in diabetic self-care an outlet for their energies.

"How can I do these painful, disgusting things?"

The routine of self-treatment can be a supremely frustrating nuisance; it can also arouse feelings of fear and disgust. Such feelings are most commonly associated with insulin injection and urine testing.

Insulin. Receiving insulin shots – and giving them to oneself – can be traumatic at first, as it was for Beth in Chapter 1. One six-year-old drew a self-portrait filled with dots, which he captioned "Pin Cushion." But people who need daily injections to survive usually get used to them pretty quickly. Typical is one man's comment that "shots are the smallest part of diabetes." Children with diabetes generally have more trouble adjusting to food restrictions than to insulin. This does not deny the discomfort, the feelings of wounding oneself, of violating oneself, of doing something "gross" which may linger on. Feelings like these may be covered up with humor or bravado. One man described himself as "shootin' up with the Big 'I'." But if a person continues to have difficulty with injections beyond the initial adjustment period, it may be a sign of some other emotional problem.

Often those who fear insulin injections the most are those who do not actually have to take them, but have reason to believe they might. People with a family history of diabetes often retain a vivid mental image of a relative's injection scars. Ironically, fear and distaste tend to be bigger problems for people with type 2 diabetes than for those with type 1. Physicians find that type 2 patients, who need to take insulin temporarily, frequently have difficulty adjusting to the routine – until a heart attack or other serious complication puts this difficulty in perspective.

If you have type 2 diabetes, or are close to someone who does, you may be able to recognize your own feelings about the prospect of insulin injections in these quotations:

"If they'd told me I had to shoot insulin I think I'd rather have died. I might well have ignored it just as I did the other kind of diabetes, rather than face the painful reality."

"To me, having to take insulin would mean a loss of control. I have an aversion to needles, too, though I suppose I could cope if I had to."

"It's not the needle I fear. It's that needing insulin would be a sign of deterioration."

"I don't know any other diabetic people like myself. The ones I know are all shooters."

Who would want to be a "shooter"? The word encapsulates a lot of emotion. Like other emotions surrounding diabetes, the fear of insulin dependence can be a prod to constructive action. But it can also have harmful consequences. It may lead a person to overcompensate (that is, to try to do too much to avoid the dreaded outcome, which is not totally within one's control anyway). The opposite extreme is denial: the possibility of becoming insulin dependent is so frightening that the person ignores it, along with what must be done to try to avoid it

People with type 2 diabetes often think about insulin shots with a sense of foreboding. Consider the aversion expressed in this account by a woman of forty who had been diagnosed sixteen years earlier. (Her story illustrates something else as well – the hopeful possibility that insulin dependence can be avoided by conscientious self-care):

Twelve years ago I went to a specialist who told me it was a "pretty good bet" that I'd need insulin sooner or later. But I haven't yet, because I've been careful about my diet and exercise. Still, the dread from those early warnings hangs over me. I wish they called what I have "low sugar tolerance" rather than "diabetes." The last sixteen years might have been different if I'd been given that less frightening diagnosis instead.

Urine testing. Urine testing runs up against a near universal taboo – a feeling powerfully summed up by Joan Hoover:

> *. . . a word or two on the fascinating subject of urine testing. When you ask a layman, for the first time, to collect the stuff and save it to play with, to turn it pretty colors, match the colors to a chart, write down the results, and do all this four times a day for the rest of his life, you had better begin by giving him a darn good reason why. You are asking him to do something he has probably considered a "no-no" since the age of two.* (Hoover, 1979)

Blood testing. Now that home blood-sugar testing has largely replaced urine testing (although urine is still used to test for ketones), feelings about blood and the pain of repeated finger pricks have become daily issues for people with diabetes, even those who do not need insulin injections. As one man with type 2 put it, "I know I don't test as much as I should. How can I when my fingers are so raw?" For this reason, testing kits that can be used on less sensitive parts of the body (such as the arms) and, in the coming years, devices that can measure blood glucose without breaking the skin at all (Klonoff, 1997) are likely to bring about major improvements in blood-sugar control.

"Did I do this to myself? to my child?"

People have a natural tendency to place blame, and about half the time they blame themselves. Guilt is a particularly tragic complication of diabetes – an unnecessary complication (strictly speaking), yet one that, given our makeup, we often have to live with. It makes sense, though, to be aware of feelings of guilt so that we can minimize their harmful consequences.

As far as we know, type 1 diabetes is not caused by anything a person does. Yet, because this disease typically strikes young children, it hits parents in a particularly painful place – their protective instinct. Parents are supposed to shield their child from harm. Diabetes penetrates the shield; ergo, the parents must have done something wrong.

Researcher M. L. Koski identified both rational and irrational guilt feelings in parents of newly diagnosed diabetic children. Rational guilt feelings are illustrated by the following example:

> *"Mother was working long hours outside of the home and did not have time to take the child to the doctor earlier."*

These, on the other hand, are irrational guilt feelings:

> *"The child was breast fed more than 1½ years; was it because of that he developed diabetes?"*

> *"Father was sick with a heart condition at the time the child was conceived; could this cause his diabetes?"*

> *"Perhaps I gave him too many sweets. I was never given sweets in my childhood, and I thought I would make it up to my children."*

> *"Why did it happen to us? What had I done to deserve this punishment?"* (Koski, 1969)

It is not surprising that the examples of irrational guilt feelings are more numerous than rational ones.

Guilt is a more complex matter in type 2 because previous behavior and life history *do* contribute to causing this disease. But that does not make it any more helpful to be moralistic toward oneself or a family member who has this form of diabetes. In the first place, hereditary and metabolic factors are also important; for example, it is much more difficult physically for some people to stay thin than for others. Second, guilt is not a good basis for remedial action. On the contrary, intense guilt is so uncomfortable that it may trigger further denial and more escapist behavior of the sort that one felt guilty about to begin with. Thus, a person who has become overweight by eating addictively may continue to go on eating binges partly to forget about previous binges. One woman who was fifty pounds overweight when diagnosed in her late thirties managed to deny her diabetes and its consequences for two years. When asked how she could thoroughly ignore her own well-being, she replied,

> My first reaction to the diagnosis was: "I did this to myself. I made myself sick." And I turned away from it because it was just too painful – the idea that this was punishment for the way I had lived.

This woman simply fit the diagnosis of diabetes into an already self-destructive life-style. It became one more reason to condemn herself, one more thing to forget by overeating.

"What will people think of me?"

Fear of the future has to do with the social as well as the physical consequences of diabetes. People who must cope with this serious chronic illness can expect to hear thoughtless remarks from neighbors, co-workers, acquaintances – remarks ranging from "Be thankful it's not leukemia" (well-intentioned, but not very helpful to, say, the parents of a two-year-old diabetic child) to "I've noticed that diabetics tend to cheat." This remark is both cruel and baseless, since it blames people for being placed in a situation where demands are made of them that most people never face. Yet it reflects a real pressure to live up to the image of a "good diabetic." A woman who has maintained excellent control for twenty-five years through careful self-monitoring and creative use of food exchanges confesses that

> One of the most embarrassing – and confining things about being known to be diabetic is that, when I'm out in public, I eat

more carefully than in fact I have to. Actually, I can eat almost any food within limits, because if you know the exchanges, you can exchange just about anything. Yet I feel as if I'm wearing a sign that reads, "She's diabetic," and people (my husband's colleagues, for instance) are looking at me and saying, "Look at her cheat!"

This pressure to conform to a stereotyped, inaccurate notion of the diabetic diet is too commonly experienced to be purely imagined. At the same time, this woman's description of the intensity and pervasiveness of such social pressure represents her own interpretation, and allowing it to influence her actions is her own choice. (These people probably pay little attention to other people's destructive habits, including even alcoholism, wife battering, and child abuse. Realizing this, she might relax in their presence.)

A person with type 1 diabetes is visibly set apart by the need to take insulin and to adhere not only to general dietary restrictions but to meal-by-meal metabolic regulation as well. The decision to join friends in a snack or a ball game can be a momentous one. In addition, there is the risk of public embarrassment in the event of a severe insulin reaction. Social stigmas can be created not only by the actual features of diabetes, but also by misinformation, as one young woman learned when two of her boyfriends asked whether they could "catch" diabetes from her.

Fortunately, the fear of being stigmatized because of diabetes is often groundless and unreal. But not always. A woman, now in her late thirties, diabetic since the age of three, recalls how she was initially rejected for admission to public school:

The town selectmen tried to keep me out of school because the teachers didn't want me. They considered me an outcast, someone who belonged in a different place. My father had to sue to get me into school. This was the worst instance of being singled out that I've experienced, and it bothered me for a long time.

One could hardly imagine a worse trauma for a six-year-old. This incident occurred in a small town in a semi-rural area where the selectmen were relatively independent of bureaucratic constraints. It occurred in the early 1950s. It seems very unlikely that it could happen today, but can we be sure?

A person with type 2 diabetes is not so visibly "different." Here there are no insulin shots or insulin reactions. But appearances can be deceiving. One man's diabetic regimen called for jogging during his lunch hour instead of eating with his co-workers. He felt that this departure from custom socially isolated him from the people he worked with. (Of course, some of his co-workers might have benefited from exercising instead of eating, but they did not have such an urgent reason to do so.) In a world where people typically socialize around food and drink, and business is often conducted over a two-martini lunch, diabetes creates some unlikely nonconformists.

"Am I still myself?"

Concern over the image others have of you reflects your own image of yourself. If you worry about whether others will accept you, then you may not fully accept yourself. Some studies have shown that diabetes represents an even greater threat to self-esteem than other chronic, incurable diseases. It is such a pervasive presence in one's life that it can be hard not to think of oneself as a "diabetic" (a label that is best avoided for this very reason), rather than as a person who, among other things, has diabetes. One man described his reaction when, in his fifties, he was diagnosed with type 2 diabetes. "I had to give up so much at one time that I was not myself for a while – not the jovial person I was." There is also, especially in type 1 diabetes, a sense of "a piece missing," a major bodily function now lost, and – in both types of diabetes – an apprehension that other parts of the body will waste away through subsequent complications. These actual and prospective losses together create a feeling of special vulnerability that can reveal itself in poignant asides. For example, a woman who developed diabetes in early childhood described herself as having been "brought up on the handouts from the Joslin Clinic," as others are brought up on the Bible.

Questions of self-esteem often focus on one's sexual image, one's attractiveness to others. The diabetic adolescent wonders, "Do I have any appeal? Will I have any dates?" Type 2 characteristically appears when sexual attractiveness is waning. Then the diabetes, itself incidental to the changes in a person's appearance, may precipitate an emotional crisis simply by crystallizing one's awareness of the aging process. Symbolic of imperfection and decay, diabetes in mid-life prompts questions like "Can I hold on to my spouse?"; "Will I ever again attract a lover?"; and "How long will I be able to satisfy my partner sexually?"

"Will I go blind? lose a leg? be disabled? disfigured?"

Two of the three diseases most feared by Americans (according to a Gallup Poll) – heart disease and blindness – are complications of diabetes. The third, cancer, serves as a metaphor for people's feelings about diabetes, as in this account by a woman who has had diabetes since childhood without complications:

> *When I developed a lump on my breast, it occurred to me that if I did have breast cancer, I wouldn't feel much different from the way I already did with diabetes. Only then did I realize the cloud of uncertainty that hangs over me.*

Or this comment from a woman who is not diabetic, but whose father died of heart failure resulting from diabetes:

> *When the doctor raised the possibility of cancer, I said, "You've hit on one of my three worst fears – cancer, disfigurement, and diabetes." Until then I hadn't realized that diabetes was one of them.*

Diabetes is seen as a sign of impending disability, disfigurement, and death because of complications that may occur years after the initial diagnosis: eye, heart, and kidney disease; problems with blood circulation; sexual dysfunction. Emotional reactions to this roulette wheel of possibilities vary. At the time of diagnosis, because the actual threat of complications is years away, both the patient and physician may pass lightly over their implications. An adolescent will commonly read off the list of complications in an American Diabetes Association handout in a rote manner and in an emotionally flat voice, like reciting the names of the presidents. This emotional distancing is useful up to a point – why worry about what might happen down the road when you're just learning how to take insulin? – as long as it doesn't get in the way of good care. On the other hand, someone who has watched a parent or other close relative develop complications (as is more common in type 2, with its higher rate of hereditary transmission) is likely to be apprehensive from the beginning. In any case, the first sign of even a mild complication can touch off an extreme upset, since it is felt to be a portent of things to come.

As with other emotional reactions, the extent to which a person dwells on the anticipation of complications depends on personality and temperament. A hard-working schoolteacher who carefully regulated her diet finally threw away the medical texts she was using for background on diabetes. She found herself imagining she had all the symptoms she read about. In general, the best preparation for the possibility of complications is careful precautions plus a realistic acceptance of uncertainty. But no amount of preparation guarantees how one will react if and when the possibility becomes an actuality. At the very least, complications intensify the preoccupation with the disease that is a normal part of diabetes. A man in his thirties, who had had type 1 diabetes since childhood, had a heart attack, loss of vision in one eye (later restored by laser treatment), and reduced sexual potency. He summed up his experience with this outburst:

This disease was attacking me everywhere. I had to diet, exercise, all those rules! Now it was attacking my sex life, my eyesight. If only I didn't have diabetes, everything would be okay in my life.

Another man in his sixties, who had lived with type 2 for a dozen years, had had open-heart surgery and (with a family history of glaucoma and blindness) had a cataract in one eye. He described this state of affairs as a "double whammy."

"Can I go on living a normal life?"

According to Freud, the two areas that define a healthy life are love and work. Diabetes, and especially its complications, pose a threat to one's ability to function normally in both areas. Thus, its diagnosis may arouse some elemental concerns about both the immediate and the long-range future – concerns about being abandoned by loved ones, being unable to provide for one's family or take care of one's children, and losing the ability to practice one's career. Many of the stories told throughout this book touch upon these fears and – in some cases – realities.

All of these fears together are powerfully evoked by the specter of severe vision loss. A computer systems designer expressed a common sentiment when he said, "Blindness is the one physical defect that can take away my livelihood." Parents of a child diagnosed at an early age may fear that disabling complications will set in before the child can even learn a career. Actual cases of severe diabetic retinopathy, while fortunately rare in proportion to all the people who have diabetes, do sometimes involve major losses in both work and family life. At the same time, while diabetic eye disease is sometimes followed by outcomes such as divorce and loss of child custody, these personal tragedies cannot be blamed on the illness and disability alone. Rather, these misfortunes place a marriage under an uncommon stress, one that would not otherwise occur. As for career disruption, blindness may end a career for which a person is otherwise particularly well suited, but it does not end the possibility of meaningful work. A blind person who could not be a nurse or a surgeon could, for example, be an effective counselor. Painting would be extremely difficult, but musical expression is relatively unimpaired.

With type 2 diabetes, dramatic disability usually does not occur until much later in life. However, a person with this disease may face painful adjustments in family life. As one woman told her type 2 diabetes group, "I feel so alone at home. No one's interested in

Shared Concerns

my problem. I just seem to get in everyone's way" (Sims and Sims, 1992). The daughter of a man with type 2 diabetes felt under pressure to work out her relationship with her father more quickly than she felt was comfortable, "while there's still time."

"Will I be left helpless?"

Two of the words that come up most frequently in interviews about diabetes are "helpless" and "control," as in "I'm afraid I'll lose control over my life." This concern is objectively remote, yet can still be subjectively vivid, at the time of onset. It can cause anxiety and depression even in a person with no physical disability. It becomes very immediate when complications actually occur or when an elderly person is diagnosed.

Fear of helplessness and dependency is aroused most dramatically by the prospect of a loss of basic functions – for example, not being able to see or to "get around" normally (after amputation). A woman whose father was diabetic draws a connection between the two when she remarks, "If I lost my eyesight I couldn't drive, and driving means freedom." Many people must feel the same way in a country that places so much emphasis on mobility.

Margery, age thirty, who has been legally blind for a year, says, "I was always so independent that it's hard even now for me to ask people's help with menus or street signs." Rather than accept prepared insulin injections from the pharmacy, she struggles to measure her own doses. Explaining that "I don't trust anybody to fill my syringes," she does trust what she concedes to be her own "guesswork":

> I use Insulgauges whose width is a measure of the number of units of insulin. The numbers are in Braille or in large print, and there is a mechanism that hooks into place when the correct number of units is drawn. Finding the stopper on the bottle is the next problem. It's hard to tell when you've drawn blood; I can see a difference in color when blood fills the syringe, but a totally blind person would not.

For Margery, demonstrating that she can exert control is as important to her sense of overall health and well-being as getting the correct dose of insulin.

The elderly often experience a frustrating loss of control in that, no matter how well they take care of themselves, complications occur anyway as other illnesses affect the course of diabetes. With diabetes complicating and complicated by other illnesses, an elderly person may really be in a dependent position, but may not have any family members to rely on. One seventy-five-year-old woman was capable of administering her own injections, and therefore of being able to live outside a nursing home, but she could not be counted on to do it regularly. Her need to depend on others was more emotional than physical.

"How long do I have to live?"

Among all the fears and concerns aroused by diabetes and its complications, death is the bottom lime. Joan Hoover captures the weight of the issue:

> *... our real, and even more unmentionable problem ... is death. You probably have not given much thought to dying or to when or how this event might come to pass. But if you are diabetic, you are constantly reminded of the possibility every morning ... it's always there, that sword of Damocles – hanging and waiting to drop.* (Hoover, 1979)

Recall the "first reactions" quoted in Chapter 1: "All I could think of was that I was going to die" (Beth, type 1); "I felt a sense of loss, a burning sensation, an 'Oh my God' feeling like when you lose your job or when a good friend dies" (Henry, type 2). Henry went on to speak of the "loss of immortality" he experienced with the diagnosis of type 2 diabetes at the age of forty. This feeling of loss can begin early in life; even a child needs to mourn. Indeed, a child has the most to lose in terms of life expectancy. When diabetes is diagnosed in middle age, the time it takes for complica-

Shared Concerns

tions to develop brings one closer to a normal life span. In the elderly, although the prospect of death is most immediate, the fear of death is least strong, since death already seems like a neighbor by the time diabetes is diagnosed.

In the words of a man in his thirties, diabetic for twenty-five years, "Two things you can't look at for a long time are the sun and your own death." People have various ways of looking away from death – in some cases by denying it, but more often by thinking and speaking of it at a distance of impersonality and intellectuality ("My life expectancy is reduced"). Various philosophies can provide consolation, such as that of traditional religion ("yea, though I walk through the valley of the shadow of death") or (for the reformed overeater) that of Alcoholics Anonymous ("I've just begun to live").

Before seeking comfort from philosophy, however, let's get the facts straight, for they, too, have a hopeful side. Diabetes does reduce average life expectancy by an average of 15 years for people with type 1, and 5–10 years for middle-aged people with type 2 (National Diabetes Data Group, 1995). Nonetheless, the gap is narrowing since the life expectancy of people with diabetes has increased. And whatever the statistical averages, no individual is necessarily doomed to a short life. One of our interviewees tells of several such cases. She has an aunt in her eighties who has been on insulin for forty years, and her doctor "sees a pair of twins with 150 years of diabetes between them." A physician cites a patient in her seventies who has been taking insulin for over forty years (and has survived breast cancer) with no major complications. This woman's blood sugar has not been particularly well controlled, although she has avoided going into diabetic comas. Here is an example from a published report:

The grandmother was diagnosed as NIDDM *[type 2] associated with obesity at age 46 yr. Control of her diabetes was achieved and maintained with weight reduction through diet therapy, and her death at age 92 yr. was attributed to cardiac failure subsequent to ischemic heart disease.* (Lawson et al., 1981)

Note that this success was achieved even though the case was diagnosed many years ago when much less was known about type 2 diabetes. One study done in 1979 (Cochran et al.) surveyed ninety-seven people who had taken insulin for fifty years or longer. The average age of the respondents was sixty-nine. The oldest of them, ninety-four, had had diabetes for seventy-nine years. Improved treatment and knowledge about self-care is lengthening the life expectancy of people with diabetes each year.

Styles of Coping

Typical Reactions

People have different ways of coping with the numerous emotional pressures brought on by diabetes. Some typical reactions follow.

Psychosomatic symptoms. Marie, age twenty-eight, was still getting used to the diagnosis of diabetes made two months earlier when she began to faint in public places, apparently from insulin reactions. She was hospitalized for testing, which revealed no abnormalities. Her physician reduced her insulin dosage to the point where insulin could not have been causing the fainting spells. "I couldn't believe it," recalls Marie. "I was sure it had to be hormonal." The fainting spells stopped once Marie understood that her extreme anxiety was affecting her body chemistry.

Preoccupation. Sylvia, age thirty-five, seemed to be monitoring her diabetes every minute of the day. In characteristically pleasant tones she always managed to direct the conversation to her blood sugar, food exchanges, and so forth.

Withdrawal. Eric, age seven, felt ashamed to have diabetes. He didn't tell anyone in school about it. During his school years he stayed out of active sports, didn't make close friends, and usually came home right after school. He did not appear to have much of a sense of humor. When he got to college he began drinking alone in bars.

Smiling depression. Steve, age fifteen, was the perfect all-American boy as he strode through the high school corridors. He spoke nonchalantly of his diabetes, but shrugged off all efforts by his parents to help him "open up" about his feelings.

Overcompensation. Ron, age forty-two, was always either pushing hard in the office to achieve career goals or out on the jogging path. "You mean everybody doesn't run a half-marathon a day?" he asked. He seemed to be racing against time – to log his lifetime quota of miles.

Intellectualization. Joan, age twenty-three, was a walking actuarial table when it came to diabetes. She knew all the food exchanges from memory and delighted in the intricacies of hemoglobin monitoring. "Let's see," she would muse, "if exercising takes an hour a day, and if regular exercise increases my life expectancy by eight years, will I gain or lose time overall by exercising?"

Self-destructive recklessness. Jerome, age twenty-six, smoked cigarettes and went on drinking binges. Sometimes he went out late at night and drove down a lonely highway at ninety miles per hour. When his sister pointed out that his behavior might have something to do with the chronic tiredness he was beginning to feel, he said, "What the hell – life is a crap game for me, anyway."

All of these are, up to a point, natural, normal reactions. They represent the many ways people cope with an abnormal situation. It is important, however, to be conscious of these emotional stances so as not to take them to harmful extremes. As time goes on, we do not have to remain stereotypes of ourselves by behaving in a rigidly routine fashion. Instead we can add a note of reason and good sense to our instinctive reactions. What we then have is a positive style of coping.

Rising to the occasion. No one is immune to emotional variations, especially with diabetes. There are times when we feel depressed, frustrated, or angry. But we also have a reserve of emotional strength, accessible once we accept diabetes as a "given" and go on from there. In mastering the challenge to live fully with diabetes, we may grow to be more effective in other dealings with the world than we would otherwise be.

Common Personality Types

As a benchmark for self-evaluation, it may be useful to keep in mind the three major personality types that psychologists have associated with different styles of coping with diabetes. None is, in itself, either good or bad. It is simply that, if you recognize yourself in one of these descriptions, you can be more conscious of who you are and thus not be at the mercy of long-ingrained, ill-understood patterns of behavior. Any one of these personality styles can be healthy or unhealthy, depending on how well it meets the requirements of a particular situation.

The dependent personality. The dependent person is used to being taken care of by others – parents, spouses, physicians, and so forth. This is a person who does not really mind being in the hospital and does not usually get into conflicts with doctors and nurses, but may not reliably practice good self-management at home. The dependent person's lapses in self-care may consciously or unconsciously serve the purpose of necessitating attention and care from others. Often this care is readily forthcoming, because the family structure (even before the diabetes) has assigned the patient a dependent role and other family members a caretaking role.

The orderly, controlled personality. In some ways this is the opposite of the dependent personality. The orderly, controlled person is restless and frustrated when on bed rest (especially in the hospital), but quite conscientious about self-management. This person often adapts well to diabetes, which is taken up as a challenge to his or her organizational skill and mastery of detail. There are, however, a couple of pitfalls here. First, a person who intellectualizes may get sidetracked into reading vast amounts of literature on diabetes and analyzing and debating the contents, at the expense of actually following simple principles of good care. Second, a person who sets up an orderly, controlled universe may feel deeply betrayed when the real world doesn't conform to the pattern, as when complications develop despite rigorous self-management.

The dramatic personality. While dependent personalities know that they want to be taken care of, and orderly, controlled personalities know that they do not, the dramatic personality is just not sure. This energetic, gregarious person typically copes with diabetes by gathering together family and friends for support. The emotional involvements created around the dramatization of diabetes do not, however, take the simple form of dependency. Instead, they represent the working out of complicated relationships (sometimes featuring a struggle between autonomy and dependency) in the guise of treating the diabetes. Unfortunately (and unlike the case of the orderly, controlled personality), most of the vast energy expended in the process does not go directly toward better diabetes care.

These personality types are not created by diabetes. Nor do they constitute special psychological weaknesses that predispose a person to diabetes or moral flaws that people with diabetes fall prey to. Rather, they are typical human variations that are all the more visible under the stress of diabetes. It is within our power to take from each what is most valuable and give it its most constructive expression: to be connected with others without being weak and clinging, to be self-reliant without being rigid and controlling, to be outgoing without being diffuse and unfocused.

Emotions and Diabetes

We have seen some of the highly charged emotional issues that go hand in hand with diabetes. But what role do emotions play in diabetes? Is diabetes caused by emotional stress, or is it simply a source of stress? Is there such a thing as a "diabetic personality"? More research is needed to answer these questions, but enough research has been done to deflate some vexing myths, reveal interesting relationships, and raise hopeful possibilities for treatment.

First, diabetes probably is *not* caused by emotional and personality factors. Research to date has failed to confirm the notion that some people are made especially susceptible to diabetes by an emotional disorder. This idea of a "diabetic personality" is, on the basis of all that we know, a source of needless guilt and self-questioning. Diabetes afflicts a wide range of people who in other respects cover the spectrum of human variation. Some people who have diabetes, and some who do not, are abnormal in other ways (e.g., mentally ill). But most people who have diabetes are normal, well-adjusted individuals faced with an abnormal, terrifying situation. Of course, they suffer from anxiety, depression, and other forms of emotional stress. Who wouldn't, considering all the things we've listed in this chapter to worry about? These emotional problems are much more clearly a consequence than a cause of diabetes.

There is, however, one important way in which emotions indirectly contribute to causing diabetes, but it applies only to type 2. You are at greater risk for this form of diabetes if you overeat and don't get enough exercise, habits which in turn may result from emotional issues that you aren't dealing with. In this case, emotions lead to behavior, which then has consequences (such as obesity) that increase the likelihood of diabetes. There is no comparable connection between emotions and type 1. You may see a lot of emotional tensions in families with children who have diabetes, but then, you may be looking for it there and not in other families. Emotional problems in diabetic children, aside from those brought on by the disease itself, may have been caused or aggravated by the anxieties felt by parents faced with diabetes in their child. Finally, with both types of diabetes, stress may trigger the onset of the disease at a particular time even if it has nothing to do with the initial susceptibility.

Although personality and emotions do not appear to cause diabetes, they *do* influence the course of the disease. For one thing, personality and emotions obviously have a lot to do with how you cope with diabetes and how well you take care of yourself – factors that affect blood sugar levels and the development of complications. Here are some ways in which stress can have an impact on your diabetes control (Helz and Templeton, 1990; Surwit and Schneider, 1993):

First, being under stress may change the way you go about the routines of self-care, such as exercise or managing your diet/insulin balance. If you typically react to stress by overeating, for example, then stressful situations will jeopardize your diabetes care – unless you learn to change the way you respond to them.

Second, if you deal with stress by turning to the calming effect of alcohol or drugs, then you are taking in substances which (like food) alter your metabolic balance.

Third, emotions ranging from depression to anxious arousal in response to stress may lead to the production or secretion of hormones that influence the metabolism of sugar and fat. This is a *direct* effect of stress on blood sugar regulation (unlike the two listed above, which are indirect).

These findings offer hope that you can improve your diabetes control by coming to terms with the emotions that surround this illness. Indeed, research to date (while not conclusive) supports this optimism. People who exhibit a stable, healthy emotional state achieve better blood sugar control, and vice versa. It is easy to see why this is so. If you can face and master the substantial emotional challenges presented by diabetes – the feelings of anxiety, loss, depression, anger, and so forth – then both your metabolism and your behavior will be less at the mercy of wild and unproductive emotional swings. You may experience less stress and surely will cope better with stress. And you will be emotionally free to make the most sensible, constructive choices for yourself and your family.

Conversely, better metabolic control is itself satisfying and (other things being equal) leads to better emotional adjustment. Some parents and physicians have feared that making an extra effort to achieve tight blood sugar control (by self-monitoring blood glucose several times a day and injecting insulin several times a day or using an insulin pump) might be emotionally draining, especially for children. This concern appears to be unwarranted (DCCT Research Group, 1996). On the contrary, taking good care of yourself and seeing the results of successful mastery and control are psychologically rewarding. It feels good to be in control; it says that what you do matters, even when much remains uncertain. Bear in mind, though, that blood sugar levels also depend on aspects of your bodily makeup over which you have no control. By all means take pleasure in your successes, but don't be too hard on yourself for "failures" that may not be your fault at all.

If emotional stress plays an important role in diabetes and its control, them stress reduction should be incorporated into the medical treatment of diabetes. In an early study, relaxation training and biofeedback were used to help a twenty-year-old woman with previously unstable type 1 diabetes gain control of her physiological responses to stress. This treatment resulted in greater stability and a reduced insulin requirement (Fowler et al., 1976). However, an attempt to achieve similar results with a patient whose diabetes was already more stable did not work as well (Seeburg and DeBoer, 1980). Since then, stress-reduction techniques have had more consistently beneficial effects on diabetic control in type 2 than in type 1 diabetes (Helz and Templeton, 1990; Rubin and Peyrot, 1992; Surwit and Schneider, 1993). This may be because reactions to stress affect the secretion of insulin (which, of course, does not occur at all in type 1) as well as other endocrine functions important to both types of diabetes. In a major study at the Duke University Medical Center, relaxation training improved sugar metabolism in a group of patients with type 2 diabetes, in comparison with a control group hospitalized for the same period without the training (Surwit and Feinglos, 1983).

Although the mechanisms by which stress and relaxation influence the course of diabetes are not yet well understood, there is still much that you can do to take advantage of the other beneficial effects of stress reduction. At a commonsense level, you can be aware of sources of stress in your life and do what you can to reduce their impact (you cannot, of course, eliminate stress altogether). You can also ask your doctor whether stress-reduction treatment might be worth trying. Whatever you do, don't leave the effects of emotions and behavior on diabetes to chance. As Alan Jacobson, chief psychiatrist and medical director of the Joslin Diabetes Center, advises:

> It [diabetes] really is, to a great extent, a behavioral illness. Your behavior and attitudes have a great deal to do with diabetes. In that sense, anything that could set you off could potentially influence the disease. Your styles, behavior, family, its strength and weaknesses, your capacity to learn and use information – all of these factors have a profound influence on the illness. (Turkington, 1985)

At times when the emotional weight of diabetes seems overwhelming, there are several places to go for help. You can turn to a doctor, nurse, or other health professional involved in treating the diabetes. If that does not work, lay persons (either as friends or as members of a diabetes support group who have experienced similar difficulties) may be a valuable source of strength and comfort. If these resources, too, prove inadequate, psychotherapy or counseling may be called for. To make your needs and choices clearer, the chapters that follow will highlight some specific sources of stress and emotional conflict connected with diabetes and guide you in coping with them effectively.

For Further Reading

American Diabetes Association. *Type 2 Diabetes: Your Healthy Living Guide* (2nd ed.). Alexandria, VA: American Diabetes Association, 1997b.

Hoover, J. Another point of view. In B.A. Hamburg, L.F. Lipsett, G.E. Inoff, and A.L. Drash (Eds.), *Behavioral and Psychosocial Issues in Diabetes, Proceedings of the National Conference.* Washington, D.C.: U.S. Department of Health and Human Services, 1979, pp. 25–32 (NIH Publication No. 80, 1993).

Polonsky, W.H. Understanding and treating patients with diabetes burnout. In B.J. Anderson and R.R. Rubin (Eds.), *Practical Psychology for Diabetes Clinicians.* Alexandria, VA: American Diabetes Association, 1996, pp. 183–192.

Rubin, R.R., Biermann, J., and Toohey, B. *Psyching Out Diabetes: A Positive Approach to Your Negative Emotions.* Los Angeles: Lowell House, 1992.

Stages of Adaptation

4

Working through the initial emotional reactions to the diagnosis of diabetes is not something that happens in a day. Indeed, the concerns described in the previous chapter will always be present, and mastering them is a continuing, lifelong process. In this chapter we will go through the emotional stages, or signposts, that one typically meets in adapting to diabetes and accepting oneself with this disease. We will also look at what "acceptance" means to different people and in what sense it is wiser to accept than to resist (as well as vice versa!).

The Four Stages

Having diabetes represents a loss which, together with anticipated further losses, arouses feelings of grief and mourning. The process of working through and resolving these feelings is usually called "acceptance," but since some people are uncomfortable with this term we shall call it "adaptation." We can think of the process as having at least four stages: denial, anger and/or depression, bargaining, and acceptance (adaptation). Although these stages resemble Elisabeth Kübler-Ross's stages of adjustment to imminent death, there is a big difference in that, with diabetes, one is adapting to *life,* under changed circumstances.

Following the diagnosis of diabetes, as well as the times when complications appear, one may go through a series of normal negative reactions, "predictable personal crises" in the words of Dr. Alan Jacobson of the Joslin Diabetes Center (1996b). These pave the way to a renewal of personal energy, from fighting the diagnosis to fighting for a full life. Of course, not everyone goes through the stages in the same sequence (one may experience two or three of them simultaneously). But the descriptions of the stages should help you to understand your own emotional reactions and to gauge your progress in coming to terms with diabetes.

Denial

Recall the woman in Chapter 1 who said "Ha! Ha!" when her doctor suggested she might have diabetes – until the diagnosis was confirmed six weeks later. Even after the diagnosis, disbelief is a typical reaction to what might otherwise be devastating news. If you do not feel any symptoms, and if you have a healthy and successful – perhaps strong and athletic – self-image, how can you believe that you are seriously ill? Type 2 diabetes in particular is called "the closet disease" because it is so easy to conceal from oneself and others. Traditionally referred to as "mild" diabetes, sometimes reversible just by "losing a few pounds," type 2 diabetes is easy to keep "out of sight, out of mind" – especially when it evokes memories of a parent with an amputated limb or fears of losing one's job or insurance. In many homes this disease is mentioned not by its name, but in euphemisms such as "My sugar's up."

Denial may be conscious (which is called suppression) or unconscious (which is called repression). You may recognize some of your own early reactions in this list of evasions:

> He [the person with diabetes] may flatly refuse to accept the diagnosis and say, "I don't have it." He may lessen the threat by claiming to have something else. He may resort to behavior designed to avoid the issue. For example, he may forget or refuse to do the things required of him, or try to control the

treatment, or divert attention to other issues, or any number of
things designed to forestall the inevitable fact of the illness. He
may seem to accept the diagnosis, but not show an appropriate
reaction to it. He may seem to accept the diagnosis but avoid
feeling about it by such behavior as being philosophical or over-
ly concerned about the facts of the situation. (Crate, 1965)

Another tactic of denial is doctor-shopping – that is, going from doctor to doctor in the hope of getting better news.

Denial occurs not only with the fact of the diagnosis, but also with the possibility of complications. A woman who developed severe retinopathy recalls that (even after she had begun to experience vision loss) she had had the attitude that "It won't happen to me; it won't get worse than what's already happened. If you were strong enough psychologically, you could control the physical problems." This is denial not of existing reality, but of anything beyond existing reality.

Wishful thinking is also expressed in the common beliefs that diabetes is caused by happenstance rather than heredity and that diabetes can be cured (Frankel, 1975). However, during the lifetimes of some of the children who profess this mistaken belief, diabetes just might be cured. Denial in this sense can blend with hope about the future. The double-edged character of denial is strikingly apparent in this description of children aged eight to fifteen at a diabetes camp:

[T]he impact of having a serious long-term "illness" was not
fully recognized by this group of children who, on the average,
had had diabetes half their lives. This was demonstrated by
their [overwhelming] selection of diabetes [as a disease they
would prefer to have] over several far less serious conditions,
e.g., constipation, acne, or obesity. It appears that they did not
fully understand the seriousness of their condition and that they
were able to deny many of its more frightening aspects, while at
the same time accepting it as a part of their way of life. (Davis
et al., 1965)

Of course, the children were identifying with the disease that had brought them together with their fellows at this camp; they might have felt differently among non-diabetic schoolmates. Nonetheless, the story shows how denial can serve the purpose of acceptance – indeed, how denial and acceptance can seem to be one and the same – for adults as well as children with diabetes.

Denial can be harmful. A man in his fifties with type 2 diabetes said ruefully, "I think I'd have fewer problems today if I'd gone to a doctor a year earlier. Why didn't I? Because I didn't want to hear about it." But it can also be recuperative – a stage in coming to terms with a calamity that is too large to grasp all at once. A degree of denial can help a person remain calm and cool in the tumultuous early weeks of diabetes or one of its complications. On the other hand, there is such a thing as being too calm. One study found that parents of children with good diabetes control had more vivid and powerful emotional reactions to the disease than parents of children with poor control (Koski, 1969).

Anger and Depression

When the reality of diabetes begins to penetrate the shield of denial, it is only natural to get angry. In this stage the question almost everyone asks is, "Why me?" (or, in the case of a parent or spouse, "Why did it have to happen to you?"). Of course, anger isn't just felt or spoken; it is also acted out. One child stole candy and kept it in special hiding places. Another sometimes banged her head against the wall – "until I grew up and learned about other people's problems." Generally, parents are the spoken or unspoken objects of childhood anger. Even into adulthood family members and living companions bear the brunt of the diabetic person's frustrations. They are the closest listeners at hand, and who else would listen very long?

Along with the family, the object of anger most frequently is the physician, nurse, or other health professional – the messenger who brings bad news. Anger at an impersonal fate is deflected into disgruntled remarks like "They're all a bunch of quacks; they don't

Stages of Adaptation

know what they're doing." Young children typically assume that whoever diagnosed their diabetes "gave" them the disease. Although such attributions are distressing for parents and health professionals to hear, they are an entirely normal way for a child to make sense of a bewildering experience.

Another natural reaction, as the awareness of the reality of diabetes sinks in (emotionally as well as intellectually), is to get depressed (Lustman, 1994; Lustman et al., 1996). Anger and depression may represent different personal styles of reacting or simply feelings that the same person has at different times. We can see anger, depression, or both when adolescents and young adults with diabetes isolate themselves socially and lose themselves in drinking binges, reckless driving, and other self-destructive acts. One man, for example, regularly got high on marijuana as he contemplated the "sloppy death" he saw ahead of him. This is a stage in which one can do oneself permanent damage, yet it also can be a prelude to mature adaptation.

Bouts with anger or depression may occur even after acceptance of the diagnosis, whenever crises arise or the discipline seems overwhelming. Anger and depression are compounded by frustration in the face of the limits of present-day medical technology. Even the most conscientious regimen cannot control blood sugar levels as precisely as nature does in the non-diabetic person. This is in part why no one is absolutely free from the risk of complications, especially after many years with the disease. And when major disabling complications such as advanced retinopathy or loss of limbs do occur, an overwhelming sense of powerlessness – felt as either anger or depression – is a normal, understandable response.

Bargaining

Another stratagem for postponing full acceptance of diabetes is to strike a bargain with God or fate. "If I'm a 'good' patient and do what I'm supposed to," you might think to yourself, "then I won't have to worry about complications." Another variation is the bargain with the physician: "If I do everything he tells me to do, maybe he'll let me eat the desserts I want." Whether the latter bargain "works" depends on the physician, but of course it is not the physician who determines the subsequent course of the illness.

Nor, as far as we can see, is there a grand dispenser of justice who measures out consequences according to each person's virtue. To be sure, following the prescribed regimens increases the *likelihood* of staying in good health. Ultimately, though, the world is not fair. Some people get diabetes while others do not, and some people who do everything they "should" still suffer complications. Some elderly people feel a sense of betrayal when the complications catch up with them after years of good control. "I don't understand," they say. "I've always had good blood sugars." It is as if they are saying, "I've kept my end of the bargain; why hasn't God kept his?" It may or may not be a consolation to realize that the complications might have occurred much sooner in the absence of such good control.

Bargaining often arises during the early remission phase of type 1 diabetes, since the remission can seem like a reward for being "good." During this temporary respite from the injection routine it takes a very tough-minded person not to harbor wishful thoughts such as: "If I really watch my diet and say my prayers every night, maybe I won't have to take insulin again."

Acceptance/Adaptation

When it comes to diabetes, not everyone thinks that acceptance is such a good idea. Joan Hoover writes, "Acceptance as defined in the dictionary means to receive gladly, take willingly, or be favorably disposed toward. No wonder it does not apply well to diabetics." But she also says, "The best education program in the world is going to be wasted on the patient who has not accepted his disease" (Hoover, 1979). This is the dilemma of "acceptance" – to achieve realism without resignation.

Some health professionals are also sensitive to the fact that acceptance has its limits. One psychiatrist asks whether a lot of what we call "denial" should not instead be called "fearlessness." He comments:

Stages of Adaptation

If I don't have to endure diabetes, I should not ask somebody else to accept it. . . . On our children's burn unit, the nurses. . . tell us that the child who will be back in school early is the one who is difficult, angry, and uncooperative. (Cassem, 1979)

Another describes some interviews with parents of diabetic children:

[T]he mothers . . . feel that there is no such thing as acceptance. After one mother said to me, "How would you feel if you had a diabetic kid?" I understood what she meant . . . [P]erhaps we should determine at what point the diabetes stops being an issue, stops being predominant in the mind of the family members. Once it no longer is a critical issue and becomes more or less a routine in their daily lives, then, perhaps, one may speak about acceptance, but not "psychological" acceptance.
(Kovacs, 1979)

Still, there is something valuable, something positive and necessary, in the notion of acceptance. If you have reached this stage, you may recall having arrived there by a gradual process. At first, perhaps, you were ashamed. As quick as you were to spot others who had the disease, you kept a distance from them. As you experienced your loss more deeply, you may have begun to feel sorry for yourself, perhaps calling yourself derogatory names like "broken-down" and "crippled." Things began to look up as you began to draw closer to others who had diabetes. "We're different," you would explain. "Nobody who doesn't have diabetes can understand what we go through." Finally, without giving up that bond with others, you were able to see yourself as an individual – one who has diabetes, but is also special in many other ways.

Acceptance in this positive sense comes when you can say, "I have diabetes. It won't go away. Sooner or later, in one way or another, it probably will get worse. I can live fully with diabetes, but I must do so within certain limits. I am different from the way

I was before, and I am different from people who don't have diabetes, but I am still myself."

In this connection, the distinction between thinking of yourself – or someone else – as "a diabetic" and as "a person with diabetes" may seem a small one, but it can be crucial. "Diabetic" as a noun is a label, a pigeonhole, that can become a person's main identity. Call someone "a diabetic" often enough, and that person can become "a diabetic." To say "a person who has diabetes," on the other hand, puts the diabetes in perspective; it puts the person first and the disease second. This way of thinking encourages the person to take reasonable risks so as to live out his or her full potential.

Acceptance does not mean resignation. It does not mean giving up and dwelling on lost years of life expectancy, as if you had no choice about how long – and *how* – you are going to live. Acceptance means a realistic *adaptation* to the requirements of diabetes. That is, coming to terms with diabetes paves the way to exerting as much control as possible in the rest of your life. It can even sensitize you to health issues that most people ignore or take for granted, and thereby give you an added sense of purpose in living healthfully and well.

Recognizing the Stages

Don't take the four stages too literally, as if they occurred in the same set pattern for every person. Rather, use them to recognize and identify your own feelings. In that way you can go through the process of adaptation consciously, avoiding the worst extremes, while knowing that your emotional reactions are normal and shared by many others who have been in the same position.

Family members and health professionals as well should learn about these stages of adaptation, in order to understand what the person who has diabetes is experiencing. What may appear to be irrational or provocative behavior may serve the deeper purpose of helping a person come to terms with a great loss. Loved ones, too, may go through a similar process of adjustment.

Not everyone, of course, goes through all the stages in the same sequence. Some simply respond with whatever emotion or emotions they show in other crises. Some don't show denial, but go right into anger and bargaining. Others acquiesce, but in the spirit of "Okay, so I'll do what I have to," not "I accept this as part of my life." This *compliance* is a kind of outward acceptance, but is not as deep or as lasting as mature adaptation.

Throughout life you will have your good days and your bad days – days of denial, anger, bargaining, or depression – but, in the long run, acceptance and adaptation will become more and more possible.

One Person's Experience of the Stages

The stages of adaptation are all illustrated by the story of Florence, who was thirty-nine years old and fifty pounds overweight when she was diagnosed with type 2 diabetes. Florence's physician made the diagnosis on the basis of blood tests taken during a routine physical examination. Having no symptoms at the time, Florence, in her own words, "chose to ignore" the diagnosis. This was the initial stage of *denial*. Why did she act so self-destructively? In the first place, she felt guilty: "I did this to myself." This reaction was more plausible for her than for someone with type 1 diabetes, since she had probably contributed to the development of type 2 diabetes by being overweight and physically inactive. But, though it may be natural to feel guilty, it doesn't do any good. Florence's feelings of guilt were not only excessive (since her weight was not the only cause of the disease), but also harmful (since she denied the reality of the disease in order to avoid the guilt). As she put it, "It was just too painful – the idea that this was punishment for the way I had lived."

Florence's initial refusal to face the implications of the diagnosis also came about because of all the emotional energy she was pouring into a discouraging family situation. With an alcoholic husband and a child who had discipline problems in school, she was constantly under stress, and her answer to stress was to run to the refrigerator. "When I'm angry, I eat," she reported. "When I'm enjoying my home and my family, I eat, too." Florence did not have to face such large adjustments in daily living as does a person who takes insulin, but she did have to face a poignant dilemma: having to change the very habits whose persistence helped bring about the disease in the first place. How could Florence deny herself her one consolation when the rest of her life was out of order? How could she attend to her family and lose weight as well? It was easier just to avoid going to the diabetes educator to whom her physician referred her. "I didn't want to know a thing about diabetes," she recalled.

When confronted with her denial, Florence reacted with *anger,* the next stage. Chastised by her physician for her neglect of her illness, she got angry at the physician. In part she was "killing the messenger who brought bad news" – that is, directing toward the physician the anger she felt about having diabetes. Her displeasure with the physician also masked her anger at herself for not having the strength to do what she needed to do. Before long, unwilling to heed the physician's warnings or follow his instructions, she stopped seeing him altogether.

For two years Florence was able to go on denying her diabetes. Then she began to notice symptoms – fatigue, excessive thirst, blurred vision, a loss of sensation in her feet. Her anger now had several targets – fate ("Why me, after everything else I've been through?"), the physician who warned her that she might need to take insulin if she persisted in her neglect (which she took as a threat of punishment), and herself for being so "stupid." Still struggling to set her household in order, she resented this added burden. "With Al-Anon [a support group for family members of alcoholics] I was finally beginning to live, and now this happened," she said.

Florence tried half-measures to make the problem go away. She brought her vision back into focus by walking around. She ate less for a few days at a time when she felt the symptoms come on. She gave up sugar while continuing to eat pastas and other high-carbohydrate foods. These gestures aimed at placating an indifferent fate were part of the third stage, that of *bargaining,* in which a person says, "I'll be 'good' if that means I won't have to lose anything." Florence's biggest bargain turned out to be her agreeing to

Stages of Adaptation

take oral medication as prescribed by her physician. The medication was meant to be part of a comprehensive treatment regimen, but Florence took it as a substitute for any other changes in her life. In her words, "Diabinese let me continue on my merry way for another two years."

At the end of this second two-year period, the symptoms began to reappear in spite of the medication. By now Florence could not altogether deny the reality of her condition. There was no one left to be angry at except herself. Her anger, now turned in upon herself, took the form of *depression,* another station on the road to adaptation. Florence felt alone, powerless, pitiable. As she became aware that she would have to accept a fundamental reordering of her life, she felt "as if I were losing an important part of myself." That was how deeply the reflex response of opening the refrigerator door had been embedded in her very being, her sense of who she was. Although this period of depression was a difficult one for Florence, it was also a constructive one, for it was the prelude to the final stage of *acceptance,* or true adaptation.

After a final binge of denial during which she "put my diabetes on the shelf," gave up all restraint, and "ate my way from October to January," Florence became very weak. Her vision deteriorated to the point where she could not read. Even then she waited a month to see a physician. When she did, the physician said, "I hope by now you've reached the point where you're ready to accept your diabetes and do something about it." Florence replied that she had, for the loss (however temporary) of so basic a function as reading had frightened her as nothing ever had. This time she went to diabetes classes, learned about the physiology of the disease, and stuck to the necessary modifications in her diet. "What was different this time," she said later, "was that I didn't want to die."

From her experience in Al-Anon, Florence was able to adapt the Alcoholics Anonymous model of surrender to her struggle with diabetes. Her descriptions of the transformation in her life have a familiar ring to those who have heard alcoholics' accounts of the "bottoming out" that precedes sobriety:

*"This is it," I thought to myself. "I have no place else to go."
Once I saw that I was going to die, I learned that I had too
much to do in life to let that happen. I don't feel deprived of the
things I've had to let go. I've just begun to live. Before I was
nothing – somebody's wife, somebody's mother. Now I'm me.*

Florence recognizes that she ate compulsively; she was addicted to food. Through this realization she has lost twenty of the fifty pounds she needs to lose and is preparing to train as a diabetes counselor. It took her four years to go through the stages from denial to acceptance. To overcome such tenacious denial, Florence had to forge a new identity. What sounds like a joyless litany of phrases starting with "I" shows this new identity taking shape. Her acceptance of this identity saved her life. It remains for her to make another vital transition – from "living for" to "living with" diabetes.

Predictable Crises

Going through the stages of adaptation is not just a one-time thing. The progression tends to be repeated, with greater or lesser intensity, at each major landmark in one's life with diabetes. These landmarks may include:

- Initial diagnosis

- First experiences of hypoglycemia (insulin reaction) and keto-acidosis (diabetic coma)

- Pregnancy and childbearing

- Recurrent infections

- Surgery

- Appearance of long-term complications

- Disability and loss of bodily integrity

- Approach of death due to complications

Each crisis, by disrupting the equilibrium established since the previous crisis, reawakens the feelings first aroused by the initial diagnosis. With each new threat to survival (or at least to "business as usual"), you may relive the pilgrim's progress through denial, anger, bargaining, depression, and adaptation. If your memory of previous crises is a troubled one, you may have difficulty with new adjustments, new losses, new manifestations of diabetes. On the other hand, if you handled earlier life passages well, those positive experiences will bolster you in facing the next challenge.

Note that, of all the crises listed, only the first and (with type 1) the second are experienced by everyone who has diabetes. Serious complications may never occur, and death may come (as it would for anyone else) for causes that have nothing to do with diabetes.

An Illustration: Disabling Vision Loss

A particularly dramatic example of the kind of event that rekindles the shock of the initial diagnosis and the subsequent passage to acceptance is the emergence of severe retinopathy, with hemorrhages and loss of vision. Here is how a woman in her early thirties, diabetic for over fifteen years, experienced it:

> *The first time it happened it just about wiped me out. I felt terror, panic, anxiety. I was alone; my husband was working. I woke up and saw this red patch, and I immediately knew what it was because my sister had had it. You know, you wake up one morning and find your whole world changed. To this day, when I have a retinal hemorrhage, I have that adrenaline surge you go through when you think you're going to fall down the steps even though you don't.*
>
> *I called my ophthalmologist, who just said, "Stay quiet. We'll take care of you." When my husband came home and walked*

*into the bedroom, I got hysterical. He said, "We'll go to Europe;
we'll see all those things you've never seen."*

*Later that summer I had more hemorrhages. My husband
would stay with me when I was very upset; when he couldn't
take it any more, he'd just give me a lot of Valium and leave the
house.*

*Then I began to have a different type of hemorrhage, called
pre-retinal, in which the bleeding was into the vitreous instead
of just behind the retinal membrane. I could see the shadow of
the blood on the retina; it looked like ink being dropped into
water. Sometimes I could see the blood pouring in for sixteen
to eighteen hours at a time. At that time I also developed
kidney trouble, which led to a blood clotting problem. This
meant that when I hemorrhaged I had to go to the emergency
room.*

It should be emphasized that this is an unusual story. Only a small
percentage of people who have diabetes – indeed, even of those
with diabetic retinopathy – develop the more serious form of
retinopathy that leads to significant vision loss (although the risk
does increase the longer you have diabetes). Even so, this woman's
reality is a major fear that stands in the background of most
people's experience with diabetes. This fear should be tempered by
hope, even for those who do develop severe retinopathy, now that
laser treatments can in some cases restore vision. Take, for example, a woman whose initial experience of hemorrhages was as
scary and as vivid as the account above:

*I was walking along, and all of a sudden I bent down and a
blood vessel burst in my eye. My eye gushed with blood. It was
like having a shade pulled down over my eye.*

After two years of near-total blindness in that eye, her vision
cleared up with the help of twenty surgical procedures. She went
through the same grueling experience with the other eye, with the
same successful outcome.

　　　　　　　　　　　　　　　　Stages of Adaptation

In any case, it is easy to understand that severe disabling retinopathy can arouse emotional reactions every bit as vivid as those that follow the diagnosis of diabetes. Judith Oehler-Giarratana, a psychiatric nurse and diabetes counselor, tells how she and others have experienced the stages of adaptation to blindness:

I've found that the person with diabetic retinopathy enters and remains in the first stage of grieving, that of shock and denial, until he becomes legally blind or very close to it. With legal blindness, he can no longer deny his impairment and that's when the anger and depression of grieving set in.

She describes her own denial:

When I first found myself blind, I still talked and thought as a sighted person. . . . Upon becoming blind, I announced to my family, "I will never learn Braille or typing, I will never get a Seeing Eye dog, and I will never marry someone I've not seen before." I have now done all four of these things.

Even so, Oehler-Giarratana is wary of the term "acceptance":

The goal of coping with diabetic retinopathy, or any other disability, should not be acceptance or adjustment. Acceptance implies compliance or approval; adjustment suggests something final or complete. The person who is blind, just like sighted people, will always encounter new situations to which he must adapt. I believe the goal in coping with diabetic retinopathy should be what I have called "identity integration," a state in which the individual comes to terms with blindness, becomes involved in a life outside himself, and returns to the fulfillment of life goals. (Oehler-Giarratana, 1978)

Ultimately, it is not the name that matters. Whatever you call it, acceptance or integration, there is an essential emotional evolution – repeated at each crisis – that prepares the way for dealing effectively with diabetes, and with life.

To Tell or Not to Tell

Living with diabetes means different things to different people. Some fully embrace a new identity, that of a person with diabetes, while others try to minimize the importance of the disease in their lives, particularly in the image they present to the world. It's "I'm different from other people" versus "I'm the same as everyone else" – both are true; it's a question of which side of things you choose to emphasize. You can make diabetes a central focus of your daily life, mentioning it prominently in conversations and seeking out new associations among others who have diabetes. Or you can say, along with a university professor in her thirties,

> I got turned off to the diabetic world by all the complaining I heard at the hospital clinic. There's an overkill of information – it's more than you want or need to know, and it doesn't serve any useful purpose. I don't want to be a medically oriented person. I block out what isn't useful to me and go about my business. You might say I'm a "different" diabetic, in that I have too many other interests to dwell on the disease.

This attitude, unless it covers denial and neglect, can represent a healthy adaptation.

At one extreme is obsessive revelation and advertisement; at the other, concealment. With type 2 diabetes, secrecy can be tempting in delicate situations, since it is relatively easy, often more a matter of omission than of any elaborate covering of one's tracks. Type 1 is another story. For some, insulin injection is an embarrassment, and they will go to any lengths necessary to keep it hidden. For others it is as routine as swallowing a pill. A famous British diabetologist used to inject himself through his pants while lecturing to the public. The following story of a mismatched young couple, as told by the woman, is a comedy with tragic overtones:

> My boyfriend thinks of himself as an eternal victim, a prisoner of diabetes. As for me, well, I have brown hair, I'm so many

inches tall, I'm diabetic. Once the two of us took a five-hour-long train trip together. At 6 P.M. it was time for my insulin, so I took out my syringe and got ready to take my shot. My boy-friend looked shocked. "What are you doing?" he said. "We're on the train."

"I'm going to take my insulin," I told him. I mean, I'm sitting next to him, the seats are high, there's nobody across the aisle. Why should I go and do a whole big number in the bathroom when I could take the shot right through my jeans (as I often do)?

"Don't do that! Go to the ladies' room."

"Why?"

"Someone might see you."

"So what? I do it all the time. If somebody thinks I'm some kind of drug addict, I'll show them the bottle of insulin."

"Don't do it!"

"Are you ashamed? Are you embarrassed?"

"Yes I am."

I couldn't believe it. "How can you be embarrassed?"

Children often take their insulin openly and matter-of-factly. Whether they can do so depends greatly on the attitudes they learn from their parents. It is the parents who decide initially whether insulin will be administered in the presence of others or off in another room. In addition, parents who themselves have diabetes provide a model of furtiveness or openness. A child who sees his father take his shot at the dining room table before breakfast will view this act differently from one whose father locks himself in the bathroom to do it. It is the difference between a family ritual and a private one.

Our interviews are seasoned with occasional dark stories of extreme surreptitiousness: a physician discovering a bottle of Diabinese at home and thereby learning that his mother had been diabetic (type 2) for ten years; a woman who took insulin secretly (even from her husband!) until the day she died. Some of these stories may have been magnified by family folklore, but it is of interest that they become more extreme, or else more vague, as they go back in time. As we go back to the grandparents of today's young adults, we hear expressions like "One of them may have had it, but nobody ever told us the truth. The old people never told you things." This sense of guardedness and shame seems to date from the period before insulin was discovered, when "You have diabetes" was a dire pronouncement indeed. At a time when diabetes was such a grave diagnosis that in some clinics only senior physicians were authorized to make it, and when (it is said) some hospitals housed patients with diabetes on the first floor for fear they would jump out the window, no wonder people "kept it to themselves." Yet even today, despite legal protections against job discrimination (see Chapter 10), there are practical as well as personal considerations to weigh in deciding how open to be (American Diabetes Association, 1996a, p. 382).

An Illustration: Denise

The atmosphere surrounding diabetes has lightened considerably over the past two or three generations. Yet the old fears and stigmas still echo in the feelings, thoughts, and actions of the young. An example is Denise, a health systems planner. Denise lives in a modern, professional world, yet she also has lived in a secret world of apprehension and anxiety – less about diabetes (from which she has suffered no complications) than about being known as a person who has diabetes.

Denise speaks precisely and remembers precisely. She remembers her first hospitalization for diabetes at the age of six – what the doctors were like, what they said, how she learned the elementary facts about diabetes and the new rules for her life. She also remembers a stuffed animal she was given when she entered the hospital. It was her constant companion there, but when she went home she put it away and never played with it again. Nor did her parents ever ask her about it. Home was a different world from the hospital, and it seemed best to keep the two separate.

Denise's parents were kindly people who projected a quiet authority. They indicated (sometimes by implication) what they wanted her to do, but did not go into long explanations or explorations. Soon after her return from the hospital, Denise recalls, "it was announced to me" that she should not tell anyone outside the family (and close friends of her parents) that she had diabetes. Her parents wanted her to be able to live a normal life and not be treated as though she were "different." On top of that, a schoolmate had recently developed diabetes, and his mother was being blamed by some of the other parents for her "carelessness" in letting him eat too many sweets. Who needed that kind of grief? As for Denise, she was only too glad not to be tarred with the same brush as her schoolmate. It "figured," all the kids were saying, that he had diabetes, since he was such a "creep" in other ways. The last thing Denise wanted was for them – and for *him* – to think of her as being paired off with him.

It was not as easy then as it is now to observe a diabetic diet unobtrusively. Society was not as health conscious and weight conscious, nor were diet sodas as ubiquitous as they are today. There were just, in Denise's words, "those funny little bottles of strange-tasting stuff that no kid in fifty miles who wasn't diabetic would drink." Children's parties were an ordeal for Denise. She dreaded hearing what she called "the ugliest words in the language": "Can you eat . . . ?" She died a thousand deaths as those parents in whom her mother confided went through the litany: "Wait a minute – can you eat that pizza? Let's see, it's bread, cheese, tomato sauce – yes, you can eat that."

Denise's discomfort at being singled out is understandable. But so are the concern and unsureness shown by the parents who took the trouble to ask what she could eat. They could hardly be expected to take courses at the Joslin Center to learn what they should feed their young guest. Denise would have preferred to be offered desserts that she could then refuse – that is, to be treated as an adult. But since she was a child, those parents who knew she had diabetes naturally felt responsible not to give her anything that was not good for her. To them, that responsibility came before protecting her secret. Even so, Denise remembers with gratitude and affection those who did both, like the mother who put all the children's sodas in glasses with straws so that she could disguise Denise's diet soda. "Denise, I know you like root beer," she would say.

Denise devised elaborate, melodramatic routines to safeguard her secret at all costs. (When necessary, she resorted to outright lies.) At a diabetes camp where she spent her summers at the ages of eleven and twelve, she learned that other girls who had diabetes could be attractive, self-assured, and physically active like herself. This experience helped her get beyond the "creepy" image of the diabetic boy she knew in school. Yet still she kept up her secrecy, giving her best friend a false address for the summer and having her letters forwarded. "It was like a detective story," she remembers. In her struggle to avoid the stigma of public identification as a "diabetic," she became privately obsessed with that identity.

When she went to college Denise might have requested a single room for privacy. But she did not do so because she wanted to "*appear* just like everyone else." She feared she might have to explain why she wanted a single room. She felt it safer instead to confide in her roommate and swear her to secrecy on their very first day in the dorm. Her roommate responded sensitively, mentioning that her grandmother was diabetic ("Everybody's grandmother's diabetic, you know," Denise remarks). But the roommate also asked why Denise couldn't be like a classmate who joked about "shooting up." Denise replied, "To me it would be like a sex change operation." She could never tell her closest friends at college why she sometimes locked the door of her dorm room. And she passed up a newly formed diabetes group at the nearby clinic where she went as a patient because she was afraid she might run into someone she knew.

As she entered adult life, Denise found that deception generated more deception. After years of concealment, how could she suddenly say to someone, "I haven't told you all these years because I have this black hole in my otherwise well-adjusted life"? Her husband would prod her, saying, "How about if we tell the so-and-sos next time we see them?" But it was Denise's decision to make, and she held back.

What turned things around for Denise was having a baby. As she puts it, "I wasn't about to have a secret diabetic pregnancy." Clearly, though, it wasn't just this circumstance that moved her. Her pregnancy was the culmination of a long-percolating emotional growth. She had had enough of holding on to her childhood resolves about diabetes. If she was going to be responsible for another being, she had to take more responsibility for herself.

Denise's pregnancy led to some humorous revelations. When she told a long-time friend and co-worker first that she was pregnant and then that she had diabetes (all in the space of two minutes), he replied, "What else do you have to tell me? Are you gay, too?"

The story of Denise's pregnancy is told in Chapter 9. A healthy, successful experience, it gave her a new, positive sense of herself. It thus was a catalyst enabling her to break out of the confines of secrecy. The emotional high point for her came after her baby was born, when a nurse in the hospital told her, "I'm so happy when I meet a woman who's diabetic who has a healthy baby, so I can tell my daughter about it. She's diabetic, too." For the first time someone was speaking of her diabetes as something positive. Indeed, her successful pregnancy and birth with diabetes was something to boast about! Even today Denise cannot speak of this moment of communion with the nurse without being visibly moved.

Since then Denise has been speaking with old friends and associates to whom she had previously said nothing or even lied. This is not something she does casually, and indeed she still does not speak of her diabetes to people she meets at parties, but when she makes new friends she does tell them about it. Most of her friends, old and new, have responded positively, with interest and understanding. One woman, herself open and honest, became angry, seeing Denise's previous secrecy as a sign of disrespect. In this instance Denise had to mend some fences.

Sometimes Denise says to herself, "Imagine me saying this, just like what kind of car I drive." Ironically, that is also how most people (preoccupied as they are with their own lives) respond to her news. Some find her buildup unnecessarily grim and alarming, "as if I were about to tell them I had cancer." Denise probably had always overestimated the importance her condition had or would have had for others had they known about it.

Now, with "three limbs out of the closet," she can hear the word "diabetes" in conversation without feeling a thump in her heart and a clutching at her throat. Now she can even venture a joke, like (when she gave someone the wrong directions): "That's what you get when you ask a diabetic person how to get to an ice cream parlor." Most important, she can think about what she would do if her daughter developed diabetes:

> Nancy takes her inoculations well, and I'm sure she could do the same with insulin. I would teach her that diabetes isn't a negative, bad, ugly, horrible thing, and I wouldn't ask her to keep it secret. Nobody now would blame me as her mother if she got diabetes, and she wouldn't have to be afraid of what people would think of her. She wouldn't have to lie and let it dominate her life.

Denise still weighs carefully the claims of privacy against those of honest disclosure. She declined to apply for a twenty-five-year award because she did not want her name published in the Joslin Center's newsletter. But then, she explains, "Nancy is my twenty-five-year award."

Like Denise, each individual needs to find a way to be comfortable with diabetes – to define an identity that takes the diabetes into account but is not unnecessarily confining, one that is consistent with the individual's values, personal style, and practical circumstances. When one has found such an identity, it becomes easier for others to accept and respect it as well.

For Further Reading

Kübler-Ross, E. *On Death and Dying.* Collier Books, 1997.

Oehler-Giarratana, J. Meeting the challenge. *Diabetes Forecast* 31(2) (1978):31–33.

To tell or not to tell. In American Diabetes Association, *American Diabetes Association Complete Guide to Diabetes: The Ultimate Home Diabetes Reference.* Alexandria, VA: American Diabetes Association, 1996a (paperback, 1997), p. 382.

The Choices –
and the Stakes

5

Developing diabetes is like coming on stage as a character in a
morality play. Suddenly the small daily choices that most people
make without thinking ("Do I want a second helping?" "Shall I go
for a jog?") are infused with moral significance. They become
"good" or "bad." Under that kind of scrutiny a normal person
risks being labeled "bad" several times a day.

How can we separate such moralistic judgments from the real
need to take good care of ourselves? How can we reconcile personal preferences with the medical consequences of our actions?
How can we decide what sacrifices to make when those consequences – the physical "rewards" and "punishments" – are only
probable, not certain? How can we make the best possible choices
in the face of the strong feelings aroused by diabetes? How can we
know what those choices are? In this chapter we will present an
approach to these questions that can help you arrive at your own
definitions of what is "good" and "bad" for you.

Dangers of a Moralistic Approach

The language of diabetes control often has a strongly moralistic
flavor. Either you are a "good diabetic" or a "bad diabetic." The
results of urine and blood tests are also termed "good" or "bad."
Such language does not accurately describe the complex choices

involved in diabetes care. Moreover, its use can have harmful consequences. In the following paragraphs are some reasons to avoid judging behavior and outcomes – and especially people – in this way.

It turns responsibility into guilt. It leads to blaming oneself for consequences an individual may not be responsible for. For example, some "brittle" (volatile or easily upset) diabetic adolescents may have difficulty controlling their blood sugar, in part because of emotional factors largely beyond their control. It certainly makes sense to observe the rules of careful diabetes management, but that does not mean that everything that goes wrong can be blamed on "bad" conduct.

It selectively stigmatizes people with diabetes as "cheaters." Everyone is susceptible to indiscretions. In a society with an overabundance of food and food-related stimulation, the temptation to eat unwisely is almost universal. Although the consequences of overloading on dessert are more severe, a person with diabetes does not show any special moral depravity by yielding to the impulse.

It turns family members against one another. It puts one family member in a policing role over another. Joan Hoover describes this unintentional effect of well-meaning treatment programs:

[A] prominent diabetic clinic has an excellent dietary counseling program. At every session it is required that the patient be accompanied by a family member. This seems not unreasonable, yet, when I asked why, I was told that diabetics tend to lie about their eating habits, and the family members were there to verify their statements. This may make for more efficient data collection, but I hope you can see what else is happening. First, the patient finds himself immediately branded as a liar, by virtue of his disease. Second, should there be a discrepancy, the family member is forced either to testify against his relative, or, out of loyalty, to collaborate in the falsehood. And third, great tension is created within the family by establishing one member

as a resident spy upon the other. I wonder if you feel the end justifies the means. Most of us who live with diabetes would probably say it does not. (Hoover, 1979)

It turns patients against health professionals. It puts the latter, too, in a policing role (Polonsky, 1995). As long as following the regimens of diabetes care is thought of as a form of "compliance" (a term that implies external authority), the physician and other health professionals become enforcers. If, on the other hand, observing the rules is seen as an informed choice made voluntarily in one's own interest, then the health professional is free to assume the more comfortable and supportive roles of adviser and counselor.

It perpetuates the myth of the "good diabetic." The "good diabetic" always follows the rules, always cooperates with the doctor, never gets upset or depressed, and never develops complications. This myth can actually be counterproductive. If you set too high a standard and feel guilty just for having normal feelings, reactions, and imperfections, you may resort to concealment and self-deception. One young woman, for example, learned as a child to measure up to this model ("Dr. Joslin himself told me I had the most beautiful blood sugars"). Now, as an adult, she has difficulty telling her physician even about her youthful indiscretions.

The "good diabetic" myth oversimplifies a multifaceted reality: many individuals follow some parts of the regimen but not others. It is also unrealistic in that it associates good results automatically with good behavior, thus setting the stage for later disillusionment ("I did everything I was supposed to, and look what happened!").

It attaches too much significance, clinical as well as moral, to particular urine and blood test results. Urine and blood testing is essential, and frequent testing (when skillfully interpreted) can be a useful tool in improving one's blood sugar control and general health. Unfortunately, all that testing, year in and year out, can make one feel like J. Alfred Prufrock in T. S. Eliot's poem, who measured out his life "with coffee spoons." Labeling a test result "good" or "bad" obscures the fact that that result represents only one reading, one moment out of a day's or several hours' fluctuations of blood sugar. Thus, when the doctor says, "Blood sugar 120 – beautiful, you're doing very well!" those cheery words may encourage the patient to "perform" for the doctor by being "good" on the day of the examination. Worse, a judgmental attitude toward test results can lead one to avoid the judgment (one's own or someone else's) by skipping the test. It can even lead (especially in adolescents) to actual cheating – that is, substituting one person's urine for another's. Here the test result has become an end in itself rather than a means to better health.

It makes it more likely that a "slip" will turn into a "binge." People make mistakes, have weak moments, and suffer inexplicable misfortunes. If these occasional setbacks are stigmatized, they can become part of a person's self-image: "I did something bad, so I must be bad, so I guess I'll just have to go on being bad." If, on the other hand, they are interpreted matter-of-factly, they don't have to set a precedent: "Okay, this happened. Now it's up to me what happens next."

It assumes a perfectly reliable cause-and-effect relationship between blood sugar control and prevention of complications. Careful management of diabetes does help prevent complications. At least, it significantly improves the odds. But with diabetes there is no certain justice. Clinicians speak of the "Hiroshima syndrome," whereby a person who has stayed in excellent control eventually develops severe complications. Fortunately, it doesn't happen very often. But it happens enough to steer us away from moralistic interpretations of tragic outcomes. Nor should the absence of complications be taken as a visible sign of membership in the elect. Does going a certain number of years without complications mean good conduct or a good constitution? Should a person who does not have diabetes be rewarded for having a pancreas that secretes insulin?

If the easy comforts of moralistic judgment and fairy-tale outcomes are not available, does that mean there is nothing to do but trust to the winds of fate? Of course not. It means, rather, that the situation is more complex and must be seen that way. If you are a fifteen-year-old with type 1 diabetes and are told that you can no longer do half the things your friends do, how do you decide how much sacrifice is worth the cost? If you are a forty-year-old with type 2 diabetes and are told that you must break the habits of a lifetime, how do you decide how much is too much – and how much is too little? To answer these questions you need to play the odds, all the while considering your own wishes and preferences.

A Matter of Probability

After the first Surgeon General's report linking smoking with lung cancer in 1963, some smokers rationalized: since the relationship between smoking and lung cancer is statistical rather than absolute (that is, it isn't true in every case), it "doesn't matter." These smokers say, "Some people who smoke don't get lung cancer, and some people who don't smoke do get it, so there must be something else going on." Indeed, there are other causes of lung cancer, but these smokers are kidding themselves. They refuse to admit that a person who smokes is *more likely* to develop lung cancer than one who does not smoke.

The same is true for the relationship between blood sugar control and the complications of diabetes. Sure, some conscientious individuals develop complications while some who live carelessly never experience nature's retribution. But that's no reason not to take care of yourself. It's a mistake to conclude that there is nothing in between perfect justice and chaos – nothing, that is, between absolute *certainty* ("If I control my blood sugar, I won't develop complications") and absolute *uncertainty* ("My blood sugar control won't make any difference – it's all a crap game anyway").

The missing piece in this puzzle is *probability*. If you practice careful diabetes management and keep your blood sugar in good control, you are *more likely* to stay healthy and avoid severe complications. Probability may not be as firm a basis for making difficult sacrifices as certainty, but it is still very real. The book *Medical Choices, Medical Chances* (see end of chapter) explains how all medical decisions involve some degree of uncertainty;

nothing is ever completely sure. This is true whether you are dealing with diabetes, cancer, hypertension, or pregnancy and birth. Whatever you do in life, you are simultaneously making *choices* and taking *chances,* and both choice and chance contribute to the outcome. In the case of diabetes, "choice" stands for the decisions you make about diet, exercise, insulin, and other aspects of care. "Chance" stands for those organic factors, known and unknown, that put some people more at risk for complications than others, as well as those that make blood sugar control itself easier to achieve. A person who can look back on twenty-five or fifty years of good control and good health has indeed played the game of diabetes skillfully, but that person may also have benefited from the luck of the draw.

Which is more important in diabetes – choice or chance? Recent research comes down on the side of choice. For example, a major Italian study concluded that, if avoidable risk factors were removed, the occurrence of diabetic complications could be reduced by one-third (Nicolucci et al., 1996). You can decide for yourself, using the many references at the end of this chapter and at the end of the book, how critical and how feasible it is for you to maintain tight control. There has long been an observable relationship between behavior and outcome at the negative end of the spectrum. That is, if you badly neglect your diabetes care, you probably will notice the ill effects before long. Now the Diabetes Control and Complications Trial (DCCT), described in Chapter 2, has found a reliable relationship at the positive end as well. Even compared with moderately good control, tight control *does* make a difference. The more precise control that can be achieved by taking three or four shots a day instead of one or two (or by using the insulin pump), together with frequent home blood-glucose testing, is likely to be worth the price in time and trouble. Even so, given the importance of individual differences and the need to make difficult personal choices, it is neither necessary nor helpful to lay a burden of guilt on yourself on the basis of the DCCT (Polonsky, 1995).

Good preventive care and treatment are a prudent choice; neglect is reckless. But both are gambles; the odds are simply better with the one than with the other. If you choose carefully, with an eye to the risks inherent in *any* choice you make, you can spare yourself the self-recrimination that sometimes comes with hindsight. Gambling from hindsight means evaluating past decisions solely on the basis of the outcome. *Medical Choices, Medical Chances* explains why this doesn't make sense:

> *It seems natural to assume that a gamble won was a good gamble, and that a gamble lost was a bad gamble . . . The fallacy in this is that a gamble would not be a gamble if chance did not intervene. A gamble would not be a gamble if the best decision always led to the best outcome. Sometimes a wise strategy does not win. Sometimes a foolish strategy does win . . .*
>
> *In order to avoid this error, it helps to remember that past decisions were based on estimates of an uncertain situation, and that these estimates must be evaluated not only on the basis of what is known after the fact, but on the basis of what was known – and not known – before the fact.* (Bursztajn et al., 1990)

An example of hindsight reasoning: "I spent all that time testing and gave up so much that I wanted to do, and now I'm still having all this trouble." Understandable as this feeling of disillusionment is, it would be more accurate to say: "I played the odds, and I lost. Besides, if I hadn't taken care of myself I might well have suffered these complications sooner."

This was the spirit in which a young woman with rapidly deteriorating vision gambled on laser treatment. Informed that without treatment she stood to lose her eyesight within a few years, she consulted several physicians, who gave her statistical estimates of the probable outcomes of laser surgery. She reviewed these with her parents and concluded that she stood a better chance of retaining some of her vision with the treatment than without. In her case, though, the laser did further damage to her eye, and she lost the use of that eye sooner than she otherwise would have. Nonetheless, she did not repudiate her gamble. She stood by her thorough assessment of the data and took comfort from the fact that this surgery has restored the vision of many others with advanced diabetic retinopathy. At the same time, when presented with a new gamble – additional laser treatments – she turned it down.

A Matter of Value

Probability alone doesn't determine what is a good gamble for you. It tells you only what outcomes may occur and how likely each is. You then have to decide how you feel about the various outcomes. Faced with the unpalatable choice of giving up something pleasant for a somewhat probable but uncertain reward, you have to make some value judgments. Which positive outcomes are vitally important to you, and which aren't worth the effort or the risk? Which negative outcomes are you determined to avoid at all costs, and which are you willing to take a chance on? Do you like to play it safe or go for the long shot? Will you endure any inconvenience to improve the odds against a medical disaster, or would you rather experience the sure and constant (though temporary) benefit of a more "normal" daily life?

When it comes to diet, exercise, regular hours, and other lifestyle issues, then, it is not a question of "Is this allowed?" or "Is this forbidden?" or "Is this cheating?" Rather, it is a statement: "These are the choices: if you do 'X,' 'Y' becomes more likely to happen." And the question becomes: "What do you want? How much do you want it? How sure of the reward do you have to be for it to be worth the sacrifice? How do you expect to feel about this in ten or twenty years when you'll be living with the consequences?"

Specifically, most of the value judgments in diabetes care are found in the answers to the following questions:

- What do I want in the way of physical health and longevity?

- What do I want from personal relationships (family, social, intimate, casual)?

- What do I want from work?

- What do I want from leisure time?

The Choices – and the Stakes

• How much freedom and responsibility do I want?

To pose these questions seriously is to ask, "What do I have to live for?" If you think life is worth living, you will think it worth some sacrifices. If your life includes self-esteem, belonging, love, fun, intimacy, and humor, if you feel the potential for growth and accomplishment, then you will be motivated to make some prudent adjustments in your diet. In colloquial language, motivation is a matter of "what's in it for you." What is most important to you: to feel better? to live longer? to be in control? to project the image (to yourself and others) of being in control? to do what you want to do regardless of the consequences? These are the value judgments, conscious or otherwise, that define the stakes you are playing for.

Although self-management of blood sugar levels has improved in the decade of the DCCT and home blood glucose monitoring (Klein et al., 1996), most people with diabetes still do not reach the level of control that they could (Jacobson, 1996a; 1996b). Does this mean that most people with diabetes don't have very much to live for – or, in the words of a *Peanuts* cartoon, "don't *wanna* feel better"? Hardly. Rather, for a variety of reasons, people do not perceive their choices correctly. They do not understand (or admit) how susceptible they are to complications, how severe those complications are, and what the benefits of prevention and treatment are relative to their costs.

Ultimately, judgments about cost versus benefit are yours to make. However, you owe it to yourself to be aware of some of the ways people fool themselves, so that you can make choices now that you can live with years from now. It is hard to deny yourself immediate pleasure for the sake of a long-term benefit; hard to accept that there are some things you can never do again, others that you must do forever. It is easier to kid yourself, to engage in "magical" thinking, than to face what sometimes are stark alternatives. Sometimes the alternatives appear starker than they really have to be, because the flexibility in responsible coping isn't presented. The "good–bad" model may implant a sense of failure and futility; after a few "bad" tests, who would want to risk testing again?

A Matter of Value

Feelings have a lot to do with choices, for better or worse. Fear (especially of death or disability) makes it hard to be rational and to make wise decisions. Emotional support (in essence, a sharing of the uncertainty and fear) from family and friends and care providers can make the difference here. If you feel good about yourself and know that others care about you, you can make choices that respect reality instead of evading it.

Good control of diabetes is associated with a stable personality, a stable home life, and a high quality of life generally, as well as with a sense of well-being and relatively low levels of anxiety and depression (Helz and Templeton, 1990; Jacobson et al., 1994; Lustman, 1994; Overstreet et al., 1995; Rubin and Peyrot, 1992). This is not surprising. A healthy emotional state and a supportive social environment help make good control possible. Conversely, good control *feels* good, physically and emotionally. Although blood sugar control also depends on organic factors beyond your power to regulate, there is unquestionably a sense of success and accomplishment that comes from being able to chart the results of scrupulously attentive diabetes care.

There are some general approaches to psychological self-help (Ellis and Harper, 1975; Glasser, 1989; Simon et al., 1995) that seem tailor-made for the dilemmas of diabetes, in that they sum up the principles discussed here and provide guidelines for applying them. Choice becomes possible when you accept the reality of your present situation and take responsibility for your actions from that point on. Having diabetes isn't your fault; it isn't your parents' fault; it isn't the doctor's fault; it is simply the reality on which you must base your choices. The choices are still yours to make.

Watch out for irrational patterns of thought that interfere with constructive action, patterns expressed in phrases like "They should . . . ," "He must . . . ," "If only the rest of the world would cooperate with my agenda." Chapter 3 told the story of Marie, who fainted in public places from what she thought were insulin reactions. By reducing her insulin dosage her physician demonstrated that these fainting spells were caused by stress. The next time she felt faint, Marie said to herself, "This isn't 'hormones';

The Choices – and the Stakes

I'm just upset. I talked myself into this; now I'll just have to talk myself out of it. Right now I have to get where I'm going. If I want, I can be upset later." Feeling dizzy was the precipitating event, but not the cause of Marie's fainting. The cause was her *interpretation* (Ellis and Harper, 1975). Anyone can feel dizzy once in a while, but Marie was interpreting this sensation irrationally: "I'm having an insulin reaction. I may die." She stopped having the fainting spells when she substituted a rational interpretation: "I'm feeling dizzy. It's an inconvenience, but I'm not going to die. I'm busy. I can't afford the luxury of dramatizing this."

Informed choice based on probabilities and values applies equally well to type 1 and type 2 diabetes. Here are some examples of the major issues that arise with these two variations of the disease.

Dilemmas: Type 1

With type 1 diabetes, control is a matter of daily (or even more frequent) measurement and adjustment. The need to take insulin brings with it the risk of overdose and reactions, not an issue in type 2. Some of the recurring dilemmas in type 1 diabetes are these:

"How tight blood sugar control should I aim for when I am not certain of the benefits? Indeed, why should I be concerned about control at all?"

"What is the proper balance between diabetes control and other roles in life? For example, is it worth it to take several insulin injections each day when that means isolating myself that much more often from my family, friends, or co-workers?"

"The more shots I take, the more times a day I test my blood, the more I remind myself that I have diabetes. Is it all worth it?"

"If I let my blood sugar run too high, I risk complications years from now. If I try to control it too tightly, I increase the risk of

having a severe insulin reaction right now, with the possibility of loss of consciousness, brain damage, or death. Is there a happy medium, and where do I find it? Can I aim for tight control and still protect myself from acute emergencies?"

"No one will notice if my blood sugar runs a little high, but to have an insulin reaction in a public place is embarrassing. How much should I compromise my medical management for appearance's sake?"

"I'm tempted to take more insulin so I can eat more sweets, but the more insulin I take, the worse I feel."

"The fear, the uncertainty, is always there. So can you blame me if I have a little fling once in a while, just so I can forget?"

"I'm young. I have to live today. Why should I deny myself a normal life because of things that might happen years from now? It's a choice between being a 'good diabetic' and a 'good teenager.'"

The probabilistic model of medical decision making tells us that there are no simple answers to these questions. But that does not mean there are no answers, or that any answer is as good as any other. When we deal with probability rather than total certainty or uncertainty, the answers are going to be a little different for each person, and they do not remain the same as a person's life situation and needs change.

For the young adults followed for an average of six and one-half years in the DCCT, intensive treatment with the goal of tight control resulted in the following reductions in the risk of complications (DCCT Research Group, 1993):

- 76% reduced risk of eye disease (retinopathy)

- 50% reduced risk of kidney disease (nephropathy)

- 60% reduced risk of nerve disease (neuropathy)

Impressive as these improved odds are, they do not by themselves dictate individual decisions about self-care. You may differ from the DCCT study population in ways that might affect your chances of benefiting from tight control. You and your doctor may not be able to duplicate the elaborate conditions under which intensive treatment was provided in the DCCT. Finally, whatever adjusted probability estimates you may make (by calculation or by hunch) about your risk of complications, you still need to weigh the expected benefits against the costs of following an intensive regimen ("the gain against the pain").

Perhaps the most poignant – and one of the most common – "type 1 dilemma" is that of the adolescent, who, to all appearances is healthy and suffering no immediate ill effects from lapses from control, and who is set apart from his or her peers by the rituals and abstentions of diabetes. At a time in life when immediate gratification and social "belonging" are paramount, the diabetic adolescent is expected to sacrifice both for the sake of an abstraction – that is, for the sake of avoiding uncertain consequences that are at least ten or fifteen years in the future. In other words, he or she is expected to show greater emotional maturity than other adolescents.

The stresses of life affect diabetes control, particularly in adolescence (Cox and Gonder-Frederick, 1992). They also cause more difficulty for girls than for boys (Anderson et al., 1981; Kovacs et al., 1990b), although boys' blood sugar control has been found to be more sensitive than girls' to family stresses over time (Jacobson et al., 1994). In past generations, girls have had to be more preoccupied with conformity than boys, more concerned with physical appearance and adequacy as a means to social success. These differences are narrowing as sex roles become less stereotyped; but, up to now, teenage girls with diabetes have had, for example, more difficulty finding boyfriends than boys with diabetes have had finding girlfriends (Koski and Kumento, 1975). Given such difficulties, girls tend to compromise their blood sugar control in the interest of other personal values. They may break the regimen by eating and drinking "what everybody else does," by keeping irregular hours that disrupt the insulin-diet balance, by taking less insulin than prescribed in order to feel more "normal," or by eating less than the prescribed diet to look attractively thin.

Our interviews provide both a forward and a backward look at this common pattern of behavior and its tragic consequences. Here is a girl of seventeen who has had diabetes for two years:

I smoke because I'm a nervous person, and I have nothing better to do. I know a girl who drinks a lot and still does well; she says she can drink instead of eating candy bars. I wish I could do that. It's so frustrating not to be able to do the things a normal person does at my age – drinking, eating certain things, partying. Sometimes I just do it. Even though they say you can feel great and be dying from diabetes, sometimes I don't even care. I figure I have plenty of time. Maybe when I get older – five or ten years from now – I'll take better care of myself, because then you don't feel like doing the same things you do when you're seventeen. I'll worry about complications then.

A woman of thirty, diagnosed at the age of thirteen, describes the life-style that preceded her becoming legally blind in her late twenties:

When I was fifteen I spent the summer traveling in Europe with a group my own age. My doctor told me to take care of myself; he warned me about all the complications. It frightened me, but not enough! I hardly slept during that trip except on the beach. I tasted everything; I especially wanted Viennese pastries. I got drunk for the first time that summer – so drunk the tour director thought I would die. I smoked marijuana, hashish, opiates, took uppers and downers, did speed to make up for the lack of sleep. Everything except mainlining; I was already taking enough injections.

This was how I lived in my teens. It was normal to do what I was doing. It would be uncomfortable, with a group of that age, to say, "I can't do that because I have diabetes." So you tell yourself, "Okay, I'll do this, and I'll take a shot to cover it."

I became more moderate in my early twenties. I found ways to fit my "wild and crazy" life-style into better control of diabetes. I thought perhaps I had settled down in time to beat the complications until my eye trouble began. Maybe I could have avoided it by being a "model diabetic," but I'll never take back what I did. The things I did in my teens and beyond – the food, the drink, the drugs, the crazy hours – were an essential part of my life. Whether or not they contributed to my loss of vision, I can only say that I wouldn't give up those experiences for anything.

These last sentences are a moving statement. The speaker denies herself the easy reflex of self-recrimination from hindsight. Instead, she stands by the gamble she took at the time, accurately recalling the probabilities that presented themselves and the value judgments she made. Nonetheless, her story is presented so that young people can consider the consequences and make a different choice. Several other women who seriously neglected their diabetes in their teens and suffered similar consequences were interviewed. Medical evidence indicates that such neglect makes loss of vision and other complications much more likely.

Dilemmas: Type 2

Type 2 diabetes often can be controlled by changing the behavior patterns (overeating and physical inactivity) that, together with genetic susceptibility, put one at risk for this condition in the first place. Better blood sugar control can, in turn, result in fewer physical symptoms, better moods, and better overall well-being for people with this type of diabetes (Van der Does et al., 1996). This is an encouraging prognosis, but doing it isn't as easy as it sounds, for it means disentangling other emotional issues from the management of diabetes and dealing with those issues in some other way. It means breaking the habits of a lifetime – habits that one learned for a reason and now must unlearn for a better reason.

Diet

In the United States food for most people is plentiful and often not presented in the most healthful form. Taken out of the context of a balanced life, it is served up anonymously in vending machines and fast-food counters. Here physical labor occupies fewer and fewer people. Alcohol is associated with solitude, boredom, and escape, rather than with family meals and rituals, and so becomes addictive. So it is with foods. When the stresses of anger, sadness, loneliness, fear, and anxiety are added to this unwholesome environment, opening the refrigerator door can become as habitual a response for one person as reaching for the bottle is for another.

For the relatively few individuals who develop type 2 diabetes without prior obesity or eating disorder, adjustment to a diabetic diet may not be difficult. For the many others who have had a special, unhealthy relationship to food, the issues are essentially the same as for the overweight person without diabetes, except that there is a more urgent reason to change. Having to exercise restraint and choose carefully from among tempting and available foods may or may not seem very difficult for a person with type 1 diabetes; it is usually traumatic for the person with type 2, who is used to eating excessively or compulsively. Although the prescribed diet may be easy to understand, motivating oneself to follow it may be anything but easy, as the case of Florence in Chapter 4 illustrates.

Treatment must include looking not only at how you use eating as a response to stress and uncomfortable feelings, but also at how you create stress in your life (while perhaps seeing it as something that "happens" to you). You also need to look at what underlying purpose being overweight may serve for you – for example, as an excuse for withdrawing from social and sexual relationships. Many helpful resources are available, including medical treatment programs and groups such as Weight Watchers and Overeaters Anonymous. However, to make good use of these resources (or to bring about positive change without them, as many do), you must undergo a profound internal revolution in the way you see your

The Choices – and the Stakes

life. You must grasp inwardly that, if you do not change, you will likely die, will suffer crippling complications, or will let your family down – or whatever future consequence seems most threatening to you. This was what Florence eventually saw.

More people than you might think, at some point in their lives, experience these revelations concerning overeating, smoking, alcohol abuse, drug addiction, and other destructive habits. They describe these moments of truth with statements like "I realized that if I kept going that way I would only do myself in" or "It suddenly hit me that every drink I took was hurting my baby." Such realizations, when they sink in, often bring about miraculous self-cures on the part of people who have resisted treatment for years (Peele et al., 1991). With diabetes, however, you may not have the luxury of waiting years for the change to occur in the natural course of your life. You may need to be more deliberate, more determined to bring about change, whether on your own or with the help of peers or professionals.

In this effort you will find support in the increasing health consciousness in society today. Although there is still an unhealthy cast to our overall social environment, with regard to food and eating habits, positive models are more in evidence now. Not only are there more – and more palatable – diet foods and drinks, but people are developing a deeper consciousness of what constitutes healthful eating and healthful living. This social evolution has made it easier for a person with diabetes (of either type) to turn down food or drink when offered and to make sensible dietary choices in the company of others.

Exercise

Exercise is essential to the treatment of type 2 diabetes (American Diabetes Association, 1997a). It begins to lower blood sugar immediately and, if kept up regularly, reduces the *insulin resistance* that causes high blood sugar in type 2 diabetes. However, these benefits cannot be felt until the person overcomes the "exercise resistance" that usually goes with overweight and a sedentary life. While many people who have been out of shape do discover at some point in their lives the value of exercise, a person who is diagnosed with type 2 diabetes is not given time for inner preparation and motivation. For this person, the need to exercise comes suddenly as an alien imposition, a chore rather than a choice.

If you are not accustomed to regular exercise, making the time and expending the energy can be as big a wrench in your daily schedule as taking insulin and testing your blood sugar. The inertia which must be overcome is physical as well as psychological, with long unused muscles adding their complaints to the general sense of upheaval and time pressure you may feel. Like other worthwhile things, exercise is likely to be painful before it becomes pleasurable. First steps are likely to be – and should be – small, but they must be followed by steady application and progress. There is a big difference between joining a health club (often pointed to with pride as a kind of personal declaration) and using the facilities regularly.

The following story typifies the mishaps in starting – and sticking to – an exercise program, even for someone who is motivated. This trim and healthy woman in her late thirties was not overweight prior to the diagnosis of type 2 diabetes sixteen years ago, nor has she been since. She is an energetic person who is as intense about exercising as she is careful about her blood sugar. Her only problem is finding an exercise she can do.

I was happiest and in my best control when I was jogging. Then I injured a knee playing tennis. A doctor specializing in sports medicine told me that jogging was the worst thing I could do for my knee joints. So I switched to swimming and was very happy with the way I adjusted to it. Then I developed osteoarthritis in my neck, so that my neck and shoulders tensed up and I was in pain a few hours after swimming. Now I walk for exercise. I've done the Jane Fonda exercises a few times, but I enjoy walking, even though it takes a lot of walking to play out the stresses. I don't like alcohol or tranquilizers, so exercise for me is the best stress reducer.

The Choices – and the Stakes

Indeed, exercise is the *natural* stress reducer, for which alcohol and tranquilizers are only substitutes. In a survey of more than 2000 adults with diabetes, their level of physical activity was the only factor within their control that predicted the quality of life they reported enjoying (Glasgow et al., 1997).

Relapse

With diet, as well as with the other life-style issues involved in the treatment of type 2 diabetes, the possibility of relapse must be allowed for – and planned for. Given that some deviation from the ideal is sure to occur, it is prudent to limit the damage in advance through some form of "relapse prevention" (Marlatt and Gordon, 1985). Relapse prevention includes avoiding combinations of circumstances in which unhealthy behavior is likely to recur (such as those producing major anxiety and stress). It also involves avoiding the moralistic attitude mentioned earlier and thinking about your behavior in such a way that a single "slip" doesn't turn into an extended "binge."

For example, if you overeat on one occasion, you may interpret it irrationally: "I did what I wasn't supposed to do. That shows that I'm a worthless good-for-nothing, powerless to control my impulses. I might as well keep breaking my diet since it seems that's what I'm going to do anyway." Or you can interpret it rationally: "For whatever reasons I gorged on lunch this one time. But that is now behind me. That lunch and whatever consequences it will have are now part of the 'givens' of my life. From here on in, though, I'm free to choose. I may not have made the best choice the last time, but I can still choose to go back to my usual healthful habits."

How you look at occasional indiscretions is an important ingredient in the success of your treatment. One woman summed it up sensibly when she said, "Once in a while I feel like hell after eating a 'no no,' but if you deny yourself that 'once in a while' you make yourself crazy." For someone with a history of compulsive eating, this insouciance may be harder to attain. A woman who had taken years to get a grip on her habit of going to the refrigerator in response to stress described how precarious she felt her new self-control to be:

> *I felt myself going back to the refrigerator, and it made me feel sick. I only ate half a sandwich, but it was half a sandwich too much. All the while I was eating it I kept telling myself it wasn't good for me. I don't know how I stopped at half. I told myself, "One sandwich is not enough, just as one drink is not enough. If I do it again, my diet is over." I think I stopped because I was afraid of what would happen if I went further. For several days after that I didn't think very well of myself.*

This woman avoided a potential binge by scaring herself with the idea that she would lose control after a second violation of her diet. The tactic worked, but it was a risky one. What if she *had* eaten the other half of the sandwich? Would she have thought herself incapable of choice at that point?

Oral Medications and Insulin

When diet and exercise alone do not bring about blood sugar control in type 2 diabetes, oral medications are prescribed to help the body make better use of the insulin it produces. When these medications do not work, insulin injections are required, either temporarily or permanently. Up to now, medicine, as practiced in the United States, has somewhat overemphasized technology and given insufficient attention to life-style issues. Some physicians prescribe insulin when oral medications would suffice, or use oral medications to treat patients who, with proper guidance, could control their blood sugar with diet and exercise. Today physicians are rapidly becoming better informed about the potential for successful treatment without medications and the value of attempting such treatment wherever possible. Nonetheless, it is still your responsibility to determine whether you are getting the best possible treatment consistent with your needs and values.

The Choices – and the Stakes

If you believe you might be able to control your diabetes with oral medication instead of insulin, or with diet and exercise instead of oral medication, ask your doctor to explain the criteria on which medical treatment was decided in your case. If you did not have a chance to try a diet-exercise regimen before being put on medications, ask your doctor why. Meanwhile, inform yourself by reading some basic sources on type 2 diabetes (American Diabetes Association, 1996a; 1996b; 1997b; Valentine et al., 1994), which indicate who is likely to benefit from the different forms of treatment and what is known about the benefits of tight control. Learn about the "second generation" of oral hypoglycemics (sulfonylureas), which can be taken in smaller doses and only once instead of two or three times a day, as well as about other oral medications such as Glucophage (metformin), that improve insulin sensitivity and can be used with or without oral hypoglycemics. (Unfortunately, the effectiveness of both kinds of oral medication slowly declines over time.) If what you read appears inconsistent with what your doctor tells you, question your doctor about it and, if necessary, seek a second opinion.

Finally, remember that diet and exercise are just as important if you are taking medications as they are if you are not. Oral medications and insulin cannot work alone, but need backup from good health habits.

A Case Study

In Chapter 4 we considered the case of Florence, who brought her addictive eating habit under control by adapting the language and techniques of Alcoholics Anonymous to her troubled relationship with food. Stanley, a forty-three-year-old scientific researcher, presents a very different variation on the same theme. To the challenge of coping with type 2 diabetes he brings a different background, a different philosophy, and a different personal style and set of idiosyncracies. His approach to diabetes, like Florence's, has strengths and limitations that reflect the person he is.

If anyone who has been living unwisely into middle age can learn quickly to make better choices, the ideal candidate would seem to be Stanley, who characterizes himself as having been "grossly overweight" when a glucose tolerance test revealed that he had type 2 diabetes. Stanley is a model of today's well-informed, actively participating medical patient. At the time of the diagnosis, he spent two hours at a university health center with his physician, who took an hour-long medical history and gave him a printed record of his blood sugar over several hours. "He was so different from other doctors – like day versus night," Stanley recalls. "He listened to me and took seriously what I said, and we figured out together what was going on." As a scientist Stanley thinks it essential to obtain accurate and complete information, and he advises others to do the same:

> Don't go to your family doctor for diabetes. Go to someone who really knows about it, preferably someone who has done some research in the area. There's no such thing as too much information. The only way you can meaningfully affect the outcome of diabetes to reduce the risks is to understand how your body works and how the disease affects it.

This advice makes obvious sense, although it may not be feasible for everyone. Physicians cannot spend two hours briefing every patient (though they can delegate this responsibility to their staff). People who do not have Stanley's professional training, and who are busy earning a living and raising a family, will not have Stanley's almost unlimited capacity to take in and process information. Stanley notes that he and his physician spent more time that first day recording data than planning treatment, and the results of his treatment thus far have been modest. He has lost sixteen pounds in the year since his diabetes was diagnosed, and some of the loss is attributable to a diuretic prescribed for high blood pressure. By his own reckoning, he has not lost enough weight to go back to the doctor he liked so much, who is in another city an hour away. Instead, he goes to a nearby clinic for tests.

Stanley explains, "I don't want any crash diet; I'm working on a life-style change. I've seen people lose sixty pounds and gain it

The Choices – and the Stakes

right back. I'd rather lose ten pounds a year and keep it off." Again, his approach is based on sound principles, although some people do lose weight quickly and keep it off.

While going about losing weight on his own terms, Stanley is critical of the medical profession:

> As far as I'm concerned, most doctors don't know what they're doing. They give out hand-me-down information with a lot of intimidating authority behind it. They tell you what to do, but not why. Their attitude is, "The less patients know the better, as long as they do what we say." Medical books for the public aren't data-based. They're just like doctors – they give you advice instead of telling you what the studies say. And they're all inconsistent. I've read three books on diabetes, and they all prescribe different diets. No wonder I haven't been able to work out my diet yet. I can't figure out what the diet should be.

Unfortunately, these observations are not entirely without foundation. Medicine has much to learn about what foods are best for diabetes. Still, it is unquestionably beneficial for a person with type 2 diabetes to lose weight, and Stanley might well concentrate on that goal. The plain fact is that limiting the kinds and quantities of food one eats is essential, even while it can be difficult, unpleasant, and frustrating. Stanley expresses understandable exasperation when he remarks, "When you go through all the things you're not supposed to eat for one reason or another, what's left? Chicken? They've got to be kidding. People I know with diabetes don't live on chicken and fish all day with a little bread and a few leafy vegetables."

Exercise is equally necessary and equally formidable ("devastating," as Stanley put it) for the person who is not used to it and who is overweight to boot. Typically, the first steps are the hardest. Stanley knows all the excuses, having used them himself at one time or another:

> "It's hard to find a time of day when it doesn't take too much time out of my schedule."

"The streets aren't safe around here, and indoor running is a hot grind."

"I got shin splints."

"Running made me dizzy."

"The chlorine in the pool hurts my eyes."

"When I exercise I lose a pound a week, and that's too much."

When Stanley began to exercise regularly he lost his appetite and felt completely exhausted in the evenings. He got past that initial discomfort and now feels more alert after running, although the pace and duration of running he believes he can safely handle are not sufficient to bring about significant weight reduction. Stanley began exercising not for fun, not out of an appreciation of its inherent benefits, but as a chore suddenly thrust upon him, a new and burdensome necessity of life. Under these conditions a certain amount of resistance is understandable.

For Stanley, the danger could be called "too much of a good thing" – namely, accumulating information. Fortunately, Stanley may be getting beyond his established habits as a result of a major event in his life, the birth of his first child. Now he has more reason to take care of himself than ever before, and he realizes it. "If I hurt myself I'm hurting my child, too," he reflects. "I want to be around to see her when she's my age." One concrete image in a person's mind can galvanize more change and motivate better choices than all the statistics that mind can hold!

Useful insights into the negative side of a dilemma like Stanley's are provided by Sidney Simon's concept of "systematic suicide." This term refers to the way people gradually, unwittingly, undramatically damage their prospects for survival in the long run by making harmful choices here and now. Even people who are otherwise well informed, people who appear to be among the world's fortunate, engage in systematic suicide for a variety of reasons (Simon et al., 1995). They do so because they

- are endowed with an enormous capacity for magical thinking.

- do not learn how to think critically.

- do not believe themselves worthy to have a better life.

- have trouble identifying what is really important to them.

- do not envision a clear future for themselves.

- do not believe they have enough to live for.

- do not identify with others who could serve as models.

- have not developed skills of self-control and communicating with others.

- do not accept responsibility for the consequences of their actions.

These observations encompass such a wide range of issues that one or more of them is bound to strike home with almost anyone. They open up questions for self-examination and psychotherapy, provide benchmarks for understanding one's past and present experience, and point to areas for restructuring one's life.

What they do not do is show how people change. Yet people do change, often by a seeming miracle, and make choices that length-en rather than shorten their lives. The hopeful note on which Stanley's case ends is by no means unique. Social psychologist Stanton Peele and his colleagues (1991) have shown that people commonly cure themselves of self-destructive habits over the course of a lifetime. They list the stages of successful self-cure.

1. Accumulated unhappiness about the addiction
2. A moment of truth
3. Changing habitual patterns of living
4. Changing from an addicted to a nonaddicted identity
5. Dealing with relapses

Stanley's vision of being with his child in forty years is one of those "moments of truth" on which a new, healthier identity can be built.

Living with Diabetes

Everyone has his or her own way of living with diabetes. One can adapt too little, endangering one's health through denial and neglect, or one can overcompensate by making diabetes the main focus of life. One can take on a "sick role," emulating the heroic therapeutic and public-relations feats of those labeled "super-diabetics," or turn one's inner life into a struggle of sin and redemption.

On the other side of the coin, giving up either the neglect that undermines good care or the overattachment to the disease that interferes with a full life may expose some uncomfortable emotions. Somewhere between the extremes, however, you may be able to find a peaceful accommodation that allows you to respect your diabetes and its needs along with your other needs. Then you can carry out the diabetic regimen seriously but flexibly, adjusting it according to the values you attach to physical health, longevity, personal relationships, work, leisure, freedom, and responsibility.

To manage diabetes with some success and satisfaction, you cannot rely on a rigid, mechanistic formula such as "If I take 'X' units of insulin, I can rely on 'Y' always to happen." The causes of your physical condition (including your blood sugar level) are always changing and are too complex to be known fully. You need to be an intuitive scientist of uncertainty and probability – experimenting daily, interpreting subtle variations according to a growing understanding of your body's resources and limits, balancing diabetes care against other priorities.

How can you carry out this continual monitoring, or at least the part of it that directly concerns blood sugar control? This is done mainly by frequent home blood glucose testing. You can get to know your body's reactions by testing a number of times daily as well as in unusual circumstances. This daily testing is supplemented by glycated hemoglobin testing (done in a doctor's office or clinic), which gives you your average blood glucose level over the past three or four months.

Another method of self-monitoring is described by a woman who has stayed in good control, with no complications and little variation in her insulin dosage, for twenty-five years:

I don't weigh food and I don't test obsessively, but in my own way I'm pretty careful. I can feel when I'm running a high sugar. It's hard to explain just how I can tell, but I trust my intuitions more than lab tests. When I feel hypoglycemic, it's an opportunity; that's when I know I can order dessert. I don't tell my doctor this, but I adjust my insulin (though only by one unit in either direction) according to how I feel. Even the modest amount of "cheating" I did as an adolescent was useful in that I learned how much latitude I had with substitutions and exchanges.

By her own testimony, and by the results she gets (including consistently normal three-month glycohemoglobin levels), this woman seems able to calibrate her own sensations in such a way as to regulate her blood sugar level. At least one study confirms that some individuals have the ability to do this. Interestingly, the particular sensations associated with fluctuations in blood glucose levels vary from person to person, so that physical cues for recognizing blood sugar variations must be individually calibrated rather than taught for general use (Pennebaker et al., 1981).

Whether self-monitoring is done by objective or subjective measures, living with diabetes is a dynamic process of adjustment and readjustment. Psychologist Stephen Jacobs has found an apt image to describe this process:

[C]ontrary to many approaches to treatment, patients who maintain the best control are not those who try rigidly to adhere to their regimen, but those who view their illness as requiring flexible (but judicious) experimentation. The view of patients in the former group might be likened to persons attempting to sit on a teetering wooden horse. The task is to remain atop, and to do so requires that they minimize sudden or extreme movements. Purposeful action toward one side or the other merely increases one's chances of falling. The view of patients in the latter group might instead be likened to persons riding a spirited mount at canter. The object is not to remain still, but to anticipate and shift with the horse's (sometimes unpredictable) movements. Only the fluid, sensitive jockey will avoid the otherwise bumpy ride. (Jacobs, 1984)

A more contemporary image is that of an airplane's inertial navigation system, which gives the pilot the continuous feedback needed for frequent adjustment of the aircraft's course.

For Further Reading

American Diabetes Association. *American Diabetes Association Complete Guide to Diabetes: The Ultimate Home Diabetes Reference.* Alexandria, VA: American Diabetes Association, 1996a (paperback, 1997).

American Diabetes Association. *Type 2 Diabetes: Your Healthy Living Guide* (2nd ed.). Alexandria, VA: American Diabetes Association, 1997b.

Beaser, R.S. *Outsmarting Diabetes: A Dynamic Approach for Reducing the Effects of Insulin-Dependent Diabetes.* Boston: Joslin Diabetes Center, 1994.

Bernstein, R.K. *Dr. Bernstein's Diabetes Solution: A Complete Guide to Achieving Normal Blood Sugars.* Boston: Little Brown, 1997.

Bursztajn, H.J., Feinbloom, R.I., Hamm, R.M., and Brodsky, A. *Medical Choices, Medical Chances: How Patients, Families, and Physicians Can Cope with Uncertainty.* New York: Routledge, 1990.

Dinsmoor, R.S. How do oral agents work? *Diabetes Self-Management* November/December 1993:46–49.

Ellis, A. and Harper, R.A. *A New Guide to Rational Living.* N. Hollywood, CA: Wilshire, 1975.

Glasser, W. *Reality Therapy.* New York: HarperCollins, 1989.

Polonsky, W.H. Besieged by the diabetes police. *Diabetes Self-Management* July/August 1995:21–26.

Rubin R.R. Rising to the challenge of tight control. *Diabetes Self-Management* January/February 1995:6–10.

Schade, D.S., Boyle, P.J., and Burge, M.R. (Eds.). *101 Tips for Staying Healthy with Diabetes (& Avoiding Complications): A Project of the American Diabetes Association.* Alexandria, VA: American Diabetes Association, 1996.

Simon, S.B., Howe, L.W., and Kirschenbaum, H. *Values Clarification: The Classic Guide to Discovering Your Truest Feelings, Beliefs, and Goals.* New York: Warner Books, 1995.

Steinburg, C. So what *is* tight control? *Diabetes Forecast* September 1993:55–58.

Steinburg, C. Tight for type II, too? *Diabetes Forecast* September 1993:61–62.

Valentine, V., Biermann, J., and Toohey, B. *Diabetes Type II and What to Do.* Los Angeles: Lowell House, 1994.

Doctors and Nurses

6

Stories about diabetes often turn out to be about doctors and nurses. Diabetes (especially type 1) brings people into frequent contact with doctors and medical staff – contact intensified by treatment aimed at achieving tight control.

> [I]ntensive treatment necessitates a more intimate working relationship than conventional therapy. Weekly telephone contact, faxing, and e-mail will often lead to stronger personal relationships and to stronger feelings as well. In this context, patients are likely to reveal more personal, emotional information and also form more intense therapeutic bonds. (Jacobson, 1996a, p. 109)

When self-care is successfully taught and measured, these bonds can be positive, satisfying ones. All too often, however, more contact simply creates more irritation and conflict. Then the doctor and patient are like an old married couple nagging at each other.

The dissatisfaction is not only on the patient's side. Diabetes calls for an active collaboration between doctor and patient. A person who has diabetes may spend an hour a week in the doctor's office, but diabetes requires attention twenty-four hours a day. Diabetes is one disease the patient treats while the doctor consults. If the doctor is too forceful, or too remote, the patient may grumble. If the patient does not assume responsibility for the treatment, the physician, forced to watch from the sidelines, may grow frustrated.

Complaints about doctors and nurses can get tiresome, but they should be not be regarded as trivial. Whether in an individual interview or a diabetes support group, grievances against health professionals can be a good starting point for facing the realities of diabetes. Feelings about other, deeper, more painful things are often deflected into gripes about the quality of medical care. Listening to those gripes (in oneself, a family member, a patient, or a fellow group member) can open doors to feelings of loss, anger, and fear that are harder to express.

Stories about diabetes are often a kind of "pilgrim's progress" from a "bad" doctor (or hospital or clinic) to a "good" one. Especially in the period just following the initial diagnosis, the doctor is seen as the messenger of bad news – news that wounds, however well it is delivered. Florence (in Chapter 4) got into a stalemate with her physician, at whom she directed her anger at herself and her fate. People often identify the physician with the illness, one reason for "doctor shopping" in the early months and years of diabetes. Once a person accepts having diabetes, it becomes easier to accept the physician as well. If you have had diabetes for some time, and if you didn't like your first doctor, think back again. Maybe you weren't in a position, emotionally, to be fair to that doctor.

On the other hand, it takes a bit of luck to find the right doctor the first time around. The first doctor you run into may actually lack the expertise or sensitivity you need. You may have to shop around to find one whose style and approach match your own. Hearing or reading about the experiences others have had with health professionals can help you identify what you like or don't like in the person who will assist you with your diabetes treatment. In this book the accounts of good and bad experiences with physicians and health care facilities illustrate different ways of practicing medicine, different ways of handling the doctor-patient relationship, and different doctors' impact on patients and families.

This chapter, while written primarily from the patient's and family's point of view, has something to say both to people with diabetes and to health professionals; it shows each how the other sees them. Health professionals can glimpse patients' concerns and expectations, and patients and families can learn what they can reasonably expect (for better and for worse) from professionals. This information is presented here not as a simulated gripe session, but to assist you in making wise choices and seeking constructive change. A relationship is a two-way street. The quality of your relationship with your doctor depends as much on you as on the doctor, for the two of you create the relationship together. If you are not satisfied with that relationship, you can create a better one, either with the same or a different physician.

Eventually, with persistence and cooperation, a relationship can be forged, in which, in the words of Linda (a woman in her late thirties who has been treated for severe retinal hemorrhages and kidney failure), "I've finally found a doctor who treats me like a human being." Mutual respect, give-and-take, clear communication on both sides – these are the qualities most often mentioned by those who are satisfied with their doctors. It takes luck to find these qualities at the outset, but with skill and effort you can find them before too long. If Linda could find them, with the serious complications she has suffered, anyone can.

Typical Complaints

Linda was not always so pleased with her medical care. Hers was a picaresque tale of misdiagnoses, incorrect decisions, personal insensitivity, and improper, irresponsible actions by physicians. Linda's grim anecdotes should be taken, not as objective descriptions, but as her *perceptions* of the physicians she has run into. As an extreme example of people's dissatisfactions with their doctors, they have a certain illustrative clarity.

My relationships with health professionals? Ha! Until recently they were a horror show. One reason now I appreciate having a doctor who talks to me and listens to me is that nobody ever did before. It was just "Take your shot" until I started having eye trouble. Then in the emergency room I was used as a visual aid for rounds. They treated me like a side show: "See the patient – 25 cents!"

Doctors never listened to my complaints or told me what was happening. They just shook their heads – it terrified me. Once when I was hemorrhaging, a doctor asked me if I had high blood pressure. I told him I didn't know, and he just dropped the matter. if he had bothered to take my blood pressure, he might have found that severe hypertension was contributing to the hemorrhages. I felt as if different parts of me were being tested, but not the whole. Whenever something came up, I didn't know who I should call: the eye man? the kidney man? the shrink?

During these years I was going up and down the East Coast to some pretty prestigious places – university and government hospitals – but the quality of care was very uneven. In New York once I came in with what I knew was an insulin reaction, but the emergency room doctor wouldn't treat me without a test, even though I had documentation that I was diabetic. That guy got chewed out by his chief. In Connecticut they refused to admit me when I had a sudden, severe glaucoma-like attack that felt like someone had stuck a red-hot poker in my eye. They gave me morphine and sent me home (I passed out in the car and had to be carried into the house). Soon afterward I was hospitalized in Maryland with a pulse of 180, blood pressure 70/30. The intern insisted it was an insulin reaction. I said, "I've been diabetic for twenty years, and I know this is not an insulin reaction. Something is wrong." I had to direct all the doctors who came in response to the code.

They kept me for three weeks of stem-to-stern biopsies and diagnosed severe malnutrition and kidney failure. They assigned me to a big diabetes man at a federal facility, who admitted me for a four-month stay. In the middle of it they told me to make a will because I was going to die within two years (this was four years ago). I mean, I was sick, but I didn't feel that sick. So they hauled in a psychiatrist to force me to accept my imminent death. After my discharge I went through the Kübler-Ross stages up to the point of joking about it (I didn't quite make it to euphoria).

*By the next summer they were saying I'd be dead by January.
"Nuts!" I replied, like the general who refused to surrender at the
Battle of the Bulge. I explained to them that they were getting me
in good control in a hospital bed, but I'd go into insulin shock
whenever I tried to live out in the world. Why couldn't they set
up more normal living conditions in the hospital, like exercise?
They told me it didn't matter; I was going to die anyway.*

*At that point someone I knew who had had diabetes for forty
years recommended a clinic in New England that had the exercise programs I wanted. The hospital in Maryland tried to stop
me from leaving, but I left "against medical advice." The New
England clinic had said they'd put me on the waiting list. "But
I'll be dead by January," I protested. They said, "Can you come
Sunday?" When I got up there a doctor examined me and
asked, "Who's the S.O.B. who told you you're going to die?"
Subsequently I had laser surgery, which improved my vision in
that eye from 20/500 to 20/100. Now I can drive a car and
read with a magnifying glass, so I guess my obituary, like Mark
Twain's, was a bit premature.*

It is difficult to untangle the real grievances here from the effects of
Linda's pugnacity, which may have contributed to the cold, insensitive treatment she experienced (we don't have the doctors' side of
the story). Later in this chapter we will look more closely at how a
jaundiced attitude toward physicians can feed into a vicious cycle
of distrust and disappointment. We will also see how Linda, who
here seems unable to utter a good word about doctors, eventually
did find a doctor she could respect.

Thus far, though, Linda's story illustrates some of the common
complaints people have about physicians and other health professionals. Among these are the following:

Missed or Inaccurate Diagnosis

Diabetes has no monopoly on this common medical occurrence.
Sometimes the diagnosis is postponed for months by a physician's

failure to do a glucose tolerance test during a physical examination; the indications for the test may not, however, have been evident at the time. Since the course of diabetes involves many subsidiary diagnoses (of ketoacidosis, hypoglycemia, and long-term complications), the possibility of missing a diagnosis exists throughout. It should also be kept in mind that the period surrounding the diagnosis is a time of emotional turmoil for patients and families, who may magnify the significance of small errors of judgment. Someone who has just suffered the blow of a diagnosis of diabetes might well imagine that "If he had spotted it six months earlier, we might have caught it in time."

Too Much Information

"They came on too heavy at the beginning" is a frequently heard lament from bewildered families. At a time when it is all one can do to adjust emotionally to the diagnosis of diabetes and learn the necessary tools for survival, diabetes education should concentrate on the basics of taking insulin and regulating one's diet. The subtleties can come later. One study found that patients interviewed immediately after a visit to the clinic remembered an average of two out of seven recommendations given them by the health care team (Page et al., 1981). Seen from the point of view of the doctor or nurse, however, this need to provide a lot of information right away is understandable. Health professionals have their own anxieties about neglecting important advice, and may feel better if everything is packed into the initial visit.

Too Little Information

Those who complain of being inundated with information don't know how lucky they are – according to another, probably larger, group of patients and families who turn to their physicians with pleas of "Harpo, speak!" Stanley, the demanding patient in Chapter 5, characterized the attitude of some doctors as "The less patients know, the better, as long as they do what we say." People complain that they are left in the dark about test results, diagnoses,

Doctors and Nurses

the rationale for treatments and instructions, and the prospect of future complications. One man, recalling his adolescence, says, "I had the feeling that they weren't telling me the whole story, just bits and pieces." Some physicians resist giving patients their medical records, to which a patient should have unquestioned access. Still, it is no picnic for the doctor to have to distinguish between patients who want more information and those who want less, especially in the emotionally charged period surrounding the diagnosis.

A woman with severe retinopathy and vision loss, who felt that her doctor always rushed her out of the examination room without adequate explanation of his findings, suggested that he make a tape, saying, "I don't know what's happening; I can't tell you why; I don't have the answer." This frustration may not be the result of the doctor's indifference, but of the fact that patient and physician alike are dealing with an inherently uncertain, frustrating condition. Retinopathy is unstable from day to day, hour to hour; thus, it generates more information than the physician can keep up with, let alone communicate to the patient. It also is a source of constant anxiety which the patient may seek to alleviate by making unrealistic demands on the physician's time and attention.

Even with these inevitable strains, a full exchange of information between doctor and patient is necessary if the person with diabetes is to be an informed patient transforming uncertainty into probabilities, as described in the previous chapter. If the physician patronizes the patient by refusing to talk or to listen, and if the patient allows this inequality and neglect to go unchallenged, then our model of effective coping with diabetes cannot be realized.

Arbitrary Prescription

Full disclosure of information goes hand in hand with an active decision-making role for the patient and family. Some patients as well as physicians still are more comfortable with an authoritarian model by which the physician dictates the treatment – no questions asked. Indeed, some people ask insistently for clear-cut instructions and criticize the doctor if these are not forthcoming. However, in today's egalitarian climate there is a growing consensus that mutuality and give-and-take, with the patient ultimately making the decisions, result in the highest quality of care and the best outcomes (Anderson, 1995; Golin et al., 1996; Greenfield et al., 1988; Rost et al., 1991). (With diabetes in particular, there is no way to avoid exercising independent judgment between visits to the doctor.)

Thus, when patients complain of doctors who instruct and prescribe without engaging the patient in the decision or even explaining the rationale, they are raising the broader issue of disempowerment. They are objecting to being denied the right and the responsibility to participate in decisions affecting their well-being. This viewpoint is expressed forcefully by Ginny, a social worker who has had diabetes almost all her life:

> *People don't just abdicate to physicians; they've never been given equal ground from which to abdicate. I used to go to one of the leading diabetes treatment centers before they had a psychosocial unit, and I found them dogmatic and ritualistic: "Do what we say, don't give us any trouble, and you'll be okay." If I chose not to go by their rules, there was nothing they could do for me. They weren't flexible enough to help me incorporate more responsible habits into my life-style. They were incapable of saying, "Now let's look at your schedule and see how we can work this in."*
>
> *The worst problems I've had have been with gynecologists – starting in my teens when a woman doctor gave me moralistic advice instead of birth control. As for male gynecologists, I'm just a body on a table to them. One told me how I'd be able to have children ("Go ahead; we'll take care of that problem") when I wasn't even interested in children; another told me to get sterilized when I was interested!*
>
> *The most petty treatment I've experienced at the hands of a physician occurred when I tried to get prescriptions for insulin so that I'd be eligible for reimbursement from the state. It would have been a break for me if the doctor had just given me the prescriptions for this over-the-counter drug that I was buying anyway. Instead, he refused to give me the prescriptions unless I*

Doctors and Nurses

came in to see him and paid for the visits. It was a power trip, a form of one-upsmanship, as if he were saying, "You need me, so you have to buy my services." That was when I switched to my present physician, with whom I get along a great deal better.

Insensitivity

Whether or not they want to participate in medical decisions, people like to be treated with respect, consideration, and compassion. In the face of the assault that diabetes represents to a person's sense of physical adequacy and integrity, no one wants to be further dehumanized by "careless handling" (i.e., callous and impersonal treatment) on the part of health professionals. Yet one often meets with physicians and nurses who are technically expert, but untrained in the skills of dealing with fellow human beings. This naiveté (more than bad will) is sometimes expressed in insensitive acts. Not surprisingly, the errors that patients and families remember most vividly are often those that occur at the time of the initial diagnosis of diabetes: announcing the diagnosis on the spot, without preparation (sometimes even over the telephone), unceremoniously telling an adolescent to "drop your drawers" for an injection immediately after the diagnosis, brushing aside a person's emotional concerns. A woman who was diagnosed in her twenties describes her doctor's inability to come to terms with the psychological ramifications of her illness:

> I have confidence in this doctor medically, but emotionally he is obtuse. He was most sensitive the first night when I was in shock and needed a physician to tell me I'd make it through. After that I hit a stone wall when I tried to share with him the range of feelings I had – my depression, helplessness, self-pity; my sense that I had betrayed my body or that it had betrayed me; my obsessive thirst for facts. He resented all my questions and my upsets. He gave me a hard time about being so "crazy" about the whole thing. Finally I told him, "You have no business comparing me with others or telling me how I should feel. I have every right to feel this way."

That these gaps in understanding continue beyond the initial period of adjustment is shown by the wry remarks people make about their (or their children's) doctors. As one woman described the professionals at a leading treatment facility, "They deal with a bleeding retina as if it were a broken fingernail." This woman might feel less dissatisfied if she understood that doctors and nurses who project this hardened image are not only under great time pressure, but also emotional pressure to protect themselves from the tragedies they see every day. The challenge for professional training is to equip caregivers to cope with these pressures while showing compassion for the patient.

Conflict Is a Two-Way Street

There is no such thing as a "bad" doctor or a "bad" patient. We can, of course, make personal value judgments about who is right and who is wrong, but they aren't very useful for improving the situation. What we *can* say is that there are *relationships* which do not work. To say that a person is bad is an opinion; to say that a relationship isn't working is an observation. We can see that two people don't get along with each other or don't work well together, and we can try to do something about it.

The Vicious Cycle of Conflict

A doctor-patient relationship that isn't working looks bad from both angles. The patient sees the doctor as dictatorial and unfeeling; the doctor sees the patient as resistant and quarrelsome. Who is right? Quite possibly both, in that they are showing each other their "bad" sides. Who provoked whom first? It is pointless to ask. In the dialectic of a deteriorating relationship, a conflict of personalities leads to ineffective treatment.

Linda's saga of difficulties with doctors was presented at the beginning of this chapter. Once, when on kidney dialysis, she heard her physician announce, "I'm going to give you testosterone."

"Huh?" said Linda. "Why?"

"Because it stimulates the production of red blood cells, which the kidneys normally take care of."

"What are the side effects? Will I grow a mustache? No offense, but I don't want a mustache."

"Linda," the physician said in an exasperated tone, "we're doing the best we can for you here. You *need* this medication."

"Look, all I want to know is, am I going to be a baritone?"

"*Linda,* why don't you just listen to me and do as I tell you?"

By this point, according to Linda, "the nurses were giggling hysterically in the background. I couldn't even see this guy, and I was yelling at him, 'You tell me what the side effects are.' Finally, he muttered and grudgingly told me that my voice might get a little lower and I might grow a mustache, but he didn't think it was likely."

The downward spiral of mutual mistrust is evident here. Was the doctor aloof because Linda was abrasive, or was she abrasive because he was aloof? Once the pattern is set, it no longer matters. Linda had a right to refuse the testosterone, regardless of the consequences. If the physician had acknowledged this right and carefully explained the side effects, Linda would have been better able to put the side effects in perspective when measured against the possibly life-saving benefits of the hormone.

In this kind of self-defeating relationship, the patient perceives the physician – perhaps all physicians – as cold, disinterested, emotionally "obtuse" (a word used by several of our interviewees). The patient retaliates by giving inadequate, misleading, or nasty answers to the physician's questions. Quick to find fault, the patient goads the physician into retreating further behind the wall of impersonal authority. The patient, lacking the nurturance provided by a supportive relationship, and inwardly unconvinced of the value of the prescribed treatment, fails to follow it or does not respond well to it.

The Physician as Parent

The moralistic "good–bad" model of diabetes self-care is tied in with a kind of relationship in which the physician is seen as an approving or disapproving parent, a role the physician may or may not actually play. Here one's relationship with one's parents becomes a model for the relationship with the doctor. A person who has been trained to seek parental approval will make an effort to produce "good" blood sugars on cue. A person who has experienced his or her parents as oppressive is likely to experience the doctor the same way – even if the doctor is not that way at all. These expectations can in turn subtly condition the physician to play the scripted role, either that of the benign, rewarding parent or that of the harsh, punishing parent. Conversely, a judgmental attitude on the part of the physician can reinforce the patient's tendency to seek approval and avoid punishment. Physicians, frustrated by their lack of control over what patients do from day to day, may turn to implicit threats of withdrawal of approval and emotional support as the only tool they have to enforce "compliance." Unfortunately, such measures reward outward performance rather than consistent self-care. They divert energy from the task at hand, which is to work out a sensible, life-long response to the requirements and consequences of diabetes.

Positive Models

Few of the people we interviewed reported having liked their first doctor. Many do like the doctor they have now (even if, in the words of one woman with retinopathy, they "had to go through seven insensitive [eye] doctors to find one sensitive one"). Among those who cite a good relationship are three of the most articulate, demanding, and dissatisfied individuals who have appeared in these pages. Stanley, the researcher in Chapter 5 who sounded as though no doctor could know enough to treat him, nonetheless spoke of his physician in generous terms: "He was so different from other doctors – like day versus night. He listened to me and took seriously what I said, and we figured out together what was going on." Respectful attention, mutual exchange, and full disclosure of findings characterized this doctor's approach. Stanley quotes him as saying. "If you listen carefully, the patient will always tell you what's wrong."

Linda, who was in and out of hospitals up and down the East Coast, and who had to fight off a premature death sentence, has "finally found a doctor who treats me like an intelligent human being." She describes how his approach differs from that of the doctors who gave orders without explanations:

After I rejected my first kidney transplant I was back in the hospital for six weeks for a second. Naturally, I feared another rejection. This doctor said, "Whenever you want a blood test, come in. You'll get over it, but as long as you feel you need it, fine." He knew how afraid I was. So what if I came in every day for a week and ended up black and blue from the blood tests. He knew I'd stop once I was reassured.

Ginny, who found most doctors authoritarian and sexist, now has one who sounds unusually realistic and respectful. He presents her with options and says, "I'll let you know as far as I can what the consequences of your choices will be, and I'll give you literature so that you can examine them further. Then it's your decision." Ginny calls this "speaking to me like an adult."

These successful relationships show that trust as well as mistrust can be mutual, and that positive as well as negative expectations can reinforce each other. Instead of a spiral of alienation and withdrawal, they show a growing momentum of confidence and comfort as two people get to know each other. Replacing the old-style relationship between doctor-as-parent and patient-as-child (where blind trust in the doctor's bag of magic turns easily to disillusionment) is a relationship between equals, two adults facing uncertainty together.

Some of the most important things a physician can do to facilitate treatment are the "simple" (actually complex and subtle) things physicians used to do before the technological era in medicine: to show caring, to take an interest in the patient as a human being, to talk and listen to the patient, and to work with the patient and family as partners in decision making. Does your doctor do these things? If not, unless you are more comfortable with an impersonal style, you may want to change the relationship or change doctors.

Just as important as the physician's personal qualities are the philosophy and procedures of the treatment program or facility. Is the human dimension included in treatment? Is someone at the clinic expert in the emotional and behavioral issues associated with diabetes, and does every patient have sufficient access to that person (or these people)? In a large treatment center, is there a psychosocial unit? In the words of one young adult, "They've known me at the clinic since I was a child. In a way, they're like my family. Yet in all that time nobody there has asked me, 'How are you doing?' Why aren't they standing by me with counselors and support groups?" Any clinic would do well to follow the lead of the Joslin Diabetes Center, which established a psychosocial unit as early as 1979 and, more recently, an Internet chat group for emotional and behavioral issues.

The need for a "human face" in treatment is most urgent in the case of adolescents facing the adjustment problems described in Chapter 5, for whom the following guidelines clearly make sense:

> [D]iscussions about independence and dependence, peer relationships, school problems, feelings of isolation and being different, changing family relationships, body image, and life as a teen-ager might be an effective approach to those adolescents who deny their illness, miss appointments, falsify urine and blood tests, "forget" to take their insulin, "miss" meals, or overeat with friends. (Sullivan, 1978)

Attention to the psychological dimension is also essential for adults with type 2 diabetes, where the persistence of the disease is tied in with the persistence of the habits that brought about its emergence. If you have this form of diabetes in part because unresolved emotional issues have caused you to be overweight, treatment that ignores those issues will have little chance of success. Psychiatrists Alan Jacobson and Stuart Hauser conclude that "[m]any factors influence the individual's coping with his or her diabetes: social support, family response, personality type, developmental level, age, and phase of diabetes" (Jacobson and Hauser, 1983). The better both you and your health care team understand this range of factors, the better your prospects for good diabetes care.

Finding the Kind of Care That Suits You

In time, people with diabetes often do find their way through the maze of the medical world and locate a congenial practitioner. Virtually everyone values honesty, respect, and trust. Fewer and fewer people are satisfied with a physician who withholds full disclosure of information. Beyond these basic principles and values, however, there is great variation in the styles of practice that people prefer. What is right for one patient or family may be wrong for another. The following are some of the different ways you can get good treatment for diabetes. You can benefit from clarifying your preferences and seeking out the options you choose.

Family Doctor versus Specialized Center

When Anne developed diabetes in her early teens, her mother continued to take her to the general practitioner in their community. Anne liked this doctor, but after a while the visits became quick and routine, "like buying gasoline." Anne wasn't getting much instruction, and she didn't feel free to ask questions in the five minutes she had with the doctor. Finally, when the family became dissatisfied with the doctor's repeated assurances that the seizures Anne was having had nothing to do with her diabetes, Anne's older brother and sister prevailed upon her mother to take Anne to a large diabetes treatment center, where she could attend classes on diabetes and where she could see a neurologist about her seizures. The doctor she had been going to said that the clinic would cost the family a good deal more without giving Anne any more information. In fact, it *was* expensive, but to Anne it was worth it. There were people available in the clinic to answer many kinds of questions, and she learned a great deal more than she had previously about diet and insulin regulation. She learned, for example, that she did not have to refrigerate the insulin she was using, which had felt cold when she injected it.

This story is typical of an age of specialized medicine. The mother was more comfortable with a family physician; her more sophisticated children advocated switching to a more "modern" treatment setting. But just as often the shift is in the opposite direction. The specialized health services that so impressed Anne were "old hat" to Penny, who had been going to a major treatment center since she was a child. There she had been treated by a prominent diabetes specialist who appeared "wan, humorless, with no smile and no bedside manner. She had the air of a researcher, and she talked only to my mother, not to me." When she was eighteen, Penny saw an internist for treatment of a minor illness. She liked him so much that she transferred to his practice for her diabetes care. What does she like about him? "He talks to me, he's friendly, and he doesn't wear whites or walk around with a stethoscope around his neck." For Penny, some small points of dress and appearance marked this physician as more accessible, more "human" than the famous specialist.

While some look at the university-based treatment center and see high-level expertise, others turn away from what they feel as coldness and impersonality. To some, going to a family doctor means not getting the latest information; to others, a family doctor stands for warmth, mutuality, and availability. A family doctor can be a heroic parent-figure whose support underlies a person's acceptance of diabetes. This double-edged reality is reflected in research on treatment effectiveness. Some studies have found that patients get better care in specialized diabetes centers than in general medical settings (Ho et al., 1997; Verlato et al., 1996). Other studies show no difference in the quality of care provided by specialist and generalist (primary-care) physicians (Greenfield et al., 1995). Unfortunately, this research reveals that much of the diabetes care provided in the United States falls short of the recommended standards of the American Diabetes Association (Marrero, 1994; Peters et al., 1996).

The parents of a four-year-old with diabetes resolved this dilemma satisfactorily by going to a pediatrician who regularly consulted an adult diabetes specialist. The family saw the diabetes specialist

Doctors and Nurses

only when the two physicians thought it advisable. This team approach combines the best of both worlds. It is, in fact, the basis of modern family practice, where the family doctor does not attempt to treat every condition singlehandedly, but also does not step aside and relinquish the patient's care if a specialist is needed. Instead, the family doctor serves as a coordinator – making the referrals, interpreting the specialists' findings and recommendations, and remaining on the scene as a familiar, reassuring presence.

Physicians versus Nurses

One way to get around the perceived aloofness of some physicians is to talk to a nurse instead. Nurses frequently have more positive emotional relationships with patients than do physicians; the patient is less likely to blame the nurse and feels more comfortable about approaching the nurse with questions. There are a number of reasons for this. Nurses do not have the aura of power that contains the seeds of disillusionment; they aren't the ones who are supposed to change the situation and make the disease go away. Nurses aren't the villains who make up the rules – i.e., restrictions. Rather, they teach and implement them. In so doing they may advocate for the patient with the physician, devise creative ways to get around the most onerous requirements, or work out palatable alternatives with a nutritionist. The nurse can set specific goals, note measurable progress, and negotiate adjustments in an atmosphere of trust and caring. A visiting nurse who comes into the patient's home gets an entirely different perspective (particularly on the patient's family life and daily habits) from that of the physician in the office. Yet the nurse is not emotionally involved in policing or adjusting to the changes in family routines – as family members are.

Anne, the teenager who left her local doctor for a well-staffed clinic, mentioned another reason for preferring to talk to a nurse. She could ask a clinic nurse "girl questions" (about sex, the effect of injection bruises on her appearance, etc.) that she would be embarrassed to ask a male physician. This distinction is, of course, diminishing as more women become doctors and more men become nurses; it does not apply to people who have physicians of the same gender. And for every five (say) Annes there is at least one Penny who gets along better with doctors than nurses. According to Penny, "My least positive medical experiences have been with nurses. When I was hospitalized in my teens, a nurse falsely accused me – in front of other patients – of sneaking candy. It was one of the most mortifying experiences of my life!"

Against this must be weighed countless other stories, like that of the parents of a newly diagnosed three-year-old who remember with gratitude one nurse they met during their child's first hospital stay. In the midst of a bombardment of instructions and criticism directed at them for being less than perfect, this nurse told them, "Hey, slow down. It's okay. Don't try to do too much in a day. Just read at your own pace and skip over whatever is too much for you. And oh, yes, I'll speak to whoever gave your child his first shot in the butt instead of in the arm."

Inpatient versus Outpatient Care

Hospitalization, when called for, has some definite advantages. It allows for intensive observation and treatment, gives the patient and family a rest from the usual chores of home care, and brings people together for mutual support. It has the disadvantage, though, of regulating a person's metabolic balance in an artificial environment. Once the person goes home – with different food, different amounts of exertion and exercise, and different stresses – insulin and dietary requirements are likely to change. More and more, physicians think it best to hospitalize a person with diabetes only for emergency stabilization. The patient is then discharged as quickly as possible, and the diet-insulin regulation is refined at home, in the person's actual living conditions. Regulating at home also reduces the sense of emergency and allows the person to experience diabetes care as a part of normal living – of wellness rather than illness.

Outpatient education is less concentrated than inpatient education but better grounded. It may take longer, but it is more likely to stick. Some people with poorly controlled diabetes have become "experts" of a sort because they are so often in the hospital being reeducated. A week in the hospital is a kind of retreat. It provides social support and a context for paying attention to diabetes control. But if it is too much fun, a person may look forward to coming back – and that is not the intended purpose. For these reasons, as well as the cost savings sought by managed care, the trend in diabetes education is toward outpatient support groups, telephone access (hotlines), and walk-in visits wherever possible. This trend is supported by research showing that the clinical advantages of outpatient care (including better blood sugar control and reduced risk of readmission to the hospital) for children newly diagnosed with diabetes outweigh the disadvantages (Charron-Prochownik et al., 1997). A drawback is that some insurers are reluctant to pay for outpatient services despite the substantial cost savings involved.

Creating a Good Relationship

What the Patient and Family Can Do

If you don't like the way your doctor relates to you and handles your care, you can do a lot more than grumble about it. If you are just beginning treatment for diabetes, or getting to know a new physician or health care team, you can do a lot to start the relationship on the right footing. In either case it is up to you to take responsibility for your end of the relationship – and, more broadly, for your own and your family's health. Here are some ways in which you can do this:

Avoid the extremes of being docile or demanding. You want to be treated as a human being and as an equal. Your doctor deserves the same respect, and so does a nurse or technician. It is not helpful to confront health professionals in an insistent, peremptory manner; nor is it in your interest to go to them with hat in hand. Good decisions can best emerge from give-and-take, not from the imposition of one person's will on another.

Decide what you want and what you need, and set goals accordingly. Every person makes a different accommodation with diabetes. You and your family should clarify your personal choices and work out with your physician a plan that honors those choices within the limits set by the disease. In this way you and your doctor will be working from a shared understanding rather than warring over "noncompliance" with unrealistic expectations.

Be concrete and specific in asking and answering questions. Do everything you can on your side to prevent misunderstanding. Come prepared with a list of questions and ask them directly, without evasion. Don't talk in euphemisms and don't accept euphemisms from your doctor. When it comes to aspects of management that you are currently dealing with yourself rather than in consultation with your doctor, keep them concrete in your mind. Ask yourself the questions *how, what, where, when,* and *why.* Between visits, keep a list of new concerns that come up. Sort them in order of priority: Do they require immediate, intermediate, or long-range resolution? Don't let yourself forget to ask questions just because you may not want to hear the answers.

Don't accept less than a full exploration of your concerns. It is your responsibility to make clear your wants and needs to your doctor and to others involved in your treatment. Don't be dissuaded until each of your concerns has been addressed – or (since not all questions can always be answered at once) until you have an agreement about when each can be addressed.

Concentrate on issues, not personalities. There is no getting around the effect the quality of the doctor-patient relationship has on the quality of treatment. Paradoxically, one thing you can do to create a better relationship is to keep the discussion focused on matters of substance. You may be aware of differences in personal style and values, but it is your choice whether you allow these to divert attention from the task at hand. If you cannot keep a personality clash from subverting treatment, find another doctor.

Take charge of your health by understanding how your body works and how it is affected by diabetes. Information pertaining to your health isn't the exclusive preserve of doctors. You can learn what you need to know in language you can understand. Somewhere between the scholar (who will not take a step without "the data") and the busy person (who "won't let medicine take over my life") is the informed consumer of health care. The more you learn, the more you can deal with your doctor as an equal partner, exercise independent judgment, and influence outcomes for the better.

Don't try to learn everything at once. It takes about twenty years to grow up and go through school. It takes time to get used to diabetes, too. If you try to learn everything at once, you are likely to get confused and not use the information effectively. Besides, much of the most useful information you will need to learn isn't found in books or pamphlets. It has to do with your individual metabolic reactions – how your blood sugar varies with changes in routine. This can be learned only over time, through trial and error.

Don't "shop around" needlessly, but do make a change when you have basic dissatisfactions. If you find yourself "doctor shopping" out of whim or perpetual discontent, remind yourself that though you can walk away from the doctor, the diabetes will walk away with you. A physician is accountable not for the diabetes, but for his or her actions. If your doctor is dictatorial, condescending, or oblivious to your feelings, you are free to go elsewhere. The doctor is in your employ, not the other way around. (Sometimes this means asking for another doctor within the same clinic, going to another institution, or even changing to another prepaid health insurance plan or health maintenance organization.)

Report negligence or improper conduct. A personality conflict, even a nasty one, has two sides; the blame should not be laid at the physician's door alone. Nor is the physician to blame for a bad outcome. On the other hand, the rare instances of real abuse – verbal, physical, sexual – or negligence in treatment should be reported to the appropriate authorities. You owe it to yourself and others to see that such conduct is brought to light.

What to Expect from the Doctor or Nurse

This section is addressed to patients and families as well as to doctors, nurses, and other health professionals. If you or a family member has diabetes, you can read this section to gain insight into what physicians and other caregivers experience. You can also use the guidelines that follow as a checklist to see how well your doctor and health care team are handling the special challenges of diabetes.

These challenges, as a rule, are not covered in the professional training of physicians and nurses. Many professionals who come into contact with diabetes at the point of diagnosis (such as a family doctor or a gynecologist serving as a woman's primary-care physician) have little specialized knowledge of the disease. When a person with diabetes comes to the hospital for treatment of another condition, the treating physician may know less than the patient about diabetes management. As a result, legitimate requests based on the patient's self-monitoring may be refused (Solowiejczyk and Baker, 1981). Even medical professionals who do specialize in diabetes are rarely trained to deal with the emotional issues covered in this book. This they must learn through experience. Some lessons that experience teaches follow.

Keeping emotional reactions separate from treatment. Even with the satisfactions that come from teaching the concrete, measurable aspects of diabetes, health professionals are deeply touched by the permanent and worsening consequences of this illness. Moreover, it can be frustrating to realize how resistant diabetes is to prevention and cure, so that one must learn other skills to be useful. The pain and frustration are real and entirely appropriate. It is healthy to acknowledge them, but it is necessary to keep them to oneself and the people with whom one shares personal feelings. If a doctor denies personal feelings, he or she may unconsciously turn away from the patient's suffering. If a nurse gets too involved in the pain, he or she may not be able to support the patient from a position of understanding, acceptance, and strength. Either way, the patient is left to suffer alone.

Maintaining an empathic, supportive relationship. A relationship built around caring and mutual trust underlies all effective medical care as well as counseling and psychotherapy. In the absence of such a therapeutic alliance, the patient may resist treatment, leading to the kind of stalemate described here by a physician:

Doctors and Nurses

Too often we discovered that, notwithstanding our efforts to work with the patient, we were perceived by him as being on the "opposite side." Disturbingly often, we found that when we said, "Believe me, this is for your own good" – the patient could not or would not believe so. We were perturbed that some of our patients saw us as demanding, and not sufficiently sympathetic; critical but not sufficiently understanding; disappointed in his failure to meet the heavy demands of a harsh chronic condition, without fully comprehending the depth and the pain of his struggle. As one young adult and long-time sufferer challenged: "What do you, doctor, really know about diabetes?" (Frankel, 1975)

In a true alliance, the patient and physician perceive themselves as being on the same side, together looking out at the difficult condition. If the patient and physician enjoy a rapport at the personal, emotional level (but with the physician remaining clearly in the role of a professional), the patient is much more likely to accept the diabetes, to contact or visit the physician when necessary, to face difficult decisions, and to follow the treatment regimen.

Balancing efficient use of time with ethical obligations to patients. Helping professionals have limited resources of time and energy. These must be wisely expended in meeting the seemingly unlimited demands of patients and families and the rigors of intensive treatment and tight control. Therefore, doctors and nurses learn to distinguish among patients who are likely to do well with or without medical attention, those whose prognosis is poor with or without treatment, and those for whom timely treatment might make a big difference. With diabetes, frequent appointments are not necessary for people who stay in good control. Nor can clinicians use themselves up by giving constant attention to those who do not respond to treatment. These guidelines do not, however, remove the helping professional's responsibility to respect each patient as an individual human being and to provide appropriate treatment within reasonable limits.

Helping with nutrition, exercise, and psychological issues as well as medical care. With diabetes, standard medical interventions are only a small part of treatment. An effective response to diabetes, like the disease itself, touches virtually every part of a person's life. Except in highly specialized medical centers, therefore, a physician or nurse needs to become familiar with many aspects of diabetes care, including life-style issues, that are not usually included in professional training.

Treating patients as whole human beings and not simply as "diabetics." As important as what one says is how one says it. Language can convey clarity, personal respect, and hope, or it can project vagueness, stereotyping, and negative expectations (Johnson, 1982). These differences in tone and emphasis reflect different ways of understanding people with diabetes. Physicians untrained in psychosocial issues sometimes attribute everything people do — including the emotions they feel and express – to diabetes. "Kids with diabetes are different," they may say, wrongly blaming the diabetes for normal adolescent developmental problems. Many generalizations we hear about "diabetics" really ought to be generalizations about *people*.

Giving concrete, specific advice. Clarity and completeness of communication (within reasonable limits) are crucial in improving diabetes self-care. Concrete, specific communications in language the patient and family can understand are essential both before the fact, in the form of clear instructions, and after, in the form of useful feedback.

One form of concrete communication available to patients and families in some clinics is behavior modification therapy, by which teaching is reinforced with systematic feedback. Here the emphasis is placed not only on providing information, but on monitoring and rewarding behavior. Among the techniques used in behavior modification are specific, unambiguous assignments, individualized skill training, cues for particular behaviors, contracts between the patient or family and the clinician, gradual approximation of the desired regimen, self-monitoring, and reinforcement of positive change (Surwit et al., 1983). Research has long been encouraging about the effectiveness of behavior modification when compared with teaching alone (Surwit et al., 1982). More recently, whether streamlined down to "brief office interventions" (Glasgow et al., 1996; Pichert et al., 1994) or expanded into a "patient empowerment" model in which patients take responsibility for their diabetes care (Anderson et al., 1995; 1996), behavioral interventions continue to show great promise (Cox and Gonder-Frederick, 1992).

Supporting both dependency and autonomy. The treatment needs to be matched to the patient. A person who is used to taking independent action may self-regulate with relative ease, while one who seeks direction from others may need more supervision. The dependent personality, the orderly, controlled personality, and the dramatic personality (as described in Chapter 3) all require treatment that works from and with – not against – their lifelong patterns of response (Kravitz et al., 1971). The patient's age also affects the equation; a child needs support both in being dependent and in outgrowing the dependency. Finally, any person who goes through the stages of adaptation to diabetes is, in a sense, like a child growing to maturity. The clinician's job is neither to argue nor to agree with the patient, but to support the patient in being in whatever stage he or she has reached. By accepting the patient's need to deny, and to be taken care of, the helping professional paves the way for the patient to accept reality and assume responsibility when ready to do so.

Being patient and refraining from giving too much information while the patient learns to cope. Some patients and families want more information at the outset than others. These differences should be respected. In general, though, it is best to let the patient set the pace by asking questions. At the beginning all information is new information. Some is more vital than the rest. An experienced social worker advises physicians and nurses, "Spoon-feed it. Let them live with it for a while – let them weather the initial shock and see that they're going to survive – before you expect them to become expert in all the subtleties."

A realistic decision-making framework. A physician or nurse can get to the heart of treatment and self-care decisions by posing questions like these to the patient and family:

"What do you want? Is it realistic?"

"What are you doing? Will it work?"

These are invaluable guidelines for people with diabetes and their families to keep in mind when away from the doctor's office: "What do I (we) want? Is it realistic? What am I (are we) doing? Will it work?"

For Further Reading

Anderson, R. M. Patient empowerment and the traditional medical model: A case of irreconcilable differences? *Diabetes Care 18* (1995): 412–415.

Bursztajn, H., Feinbloom, R. I., Hamm, R. M., and Brodsky, A. *Medical Choices, Medical Chances: How Patients, Families, and Physicians Can Cope with Uncertainty.* New York: Routledge, 1990.

Hirsch, I. B. *How to Get Great Diabetes Care.* Alexandria, VA: American Diabetes Association, 1996.

Hoover, J. Another point of view. In B. A. Hamburg, L. F. Lipsett, G. E. Inoff, and A. L. Drash, (Eds.), *Behavioral and Psychosocial Issues in Diabetes, Proceedings of the National Conference.* Washington, D.C.: U.S. Department of Health and Human Services, 1979, pp. 25–32. (NIH Publication No. 80–1993).

Katz, J. *The Silent World of Doctor and Patient.* Baltimore: Johns Hopkins University Press, 1997.

Diabetes and the Family

7

Family life, as well as dating, courtship, and all close personal relationships, is deeply affected by diabetes. At the same time, the character of family and personal life deeply affects how a person will cope with diabetes. In addition, the quality of a family's life together is perhaps the largest single factor in the metabolic stability of children, adolescents, and young adults with diabetes.

Dependency, autonomy, and rites of passage from the one to the other shape the family's response to diabetes just as to other crises. Diabetes is a crucible that reveals, focuses, excuses, intensifies, strains, and occasionally transforms the patterns people develop for getting along with one another in close quarters. It throws these patterns into bold relief, giving them more serious consequences than they otherwise might have. For this reason diabetes can mobilize a family (sometimes with the help of family therapy) to come to terms with destructive patterns that might otherwise go unnoticed and to replace them with more supportive relationships.

Many studies have shown that good family relationships are associated with stable metabolic functioning, while neglect of diabetes and "brittle" blood sugar readings often go with family friction, overprotection, or indifference. Which is the cause and which is the effect? Clearly, the cause-and-effect relationship goes both ways. Out-of-control diabetes strains family relations by stirring up feelings of frustration, inadequacy, guilt, and recrimination. Still, there is ample evidence that the way family members work together affects blood sugar control both directly (through the psychosomatic effects of stress) and indirectly (by encouraging more or less attention to self-care). Therefore, you have good reason to look at how your family is coping with diabetes and to see if you might benefit from doing things differently.

How Diabetes Affects the Family

In the words of the American Diabetes Association's manual, *Diabetes in the Family* (1987), diabetes is "an unwelcome guest who comes to stay and can threaten everyone in the family." Once this guest's baggage is deposited in the kitchen, bathroom, bedroom – all over the house – family life will never be the same. Roles may change or become more rigid; economic pressures or social isolation may threaten an established way of life. In the following sections we see how diabetes can affect a family.

A Justification for Overprotectiveness

Parents who tend to be overprotective toward their children – even into adulthood – are likely to be even more so when a child develops diabetes, which serves as a "legitimate" outlet for this impulse. Often a mother will form a closer emotional relationship with a child with diabetes than with her other children, thus encouraging dependency in the diabetic child (who takes on the role of a younger child regardless of actual birth order) and risking rejection by the others. Parents' worries about how diabetes complicates their children's development may well exceed the problem. For example, parents overestimate the effects of diabetes on their children's social life, school performance, and concentration, at least from the children's point of view.

One young man said the women he dated assumed a mothering role – for example, supervising what he ate. This was instigated by his mother, who would take the women aside and say, "He's diabetic; make sure he doesn't eat such-and-such." Irritated by this behavior, he may nonetheless have been choosing women who would carry on his mother's nurturance.

A Source of Embarrassment

A family member with diabetes – especially the head of a family – may take "shots" at the breakfast or dinner table. The others get used to the sights and smells as an accompaniment to mealtime, and it is accepted within the household. "It never bothered me," recalls the grown daughter of a man who took his injections openly, "except that I was always afraid he'd pull out the needle when we had company. If I had friends over, I'd excuse us from the table." Here what is normal among the family is seen as shameful if revealed to the outside world. This woman felt she had to be ashamed of her father. How would this affect her image of herself as she grew up? Did she think of herself as having something to hide?

A Physical Interpretation of Moods

Since variations in blood sugar level affect a person's mood, changes in mood can be a clue to physiological needs. High blood sugar can leave a person feeling tired and depressed, while low blood sugar can precipitate anger or anxiety. Because of this, some families fall into the habit of attributing *any* change in emotional state to metabolic variations. "Look how angry you are – go have some orange juice," they'll say. This habitual response can sidestep real family conflicts, even deny the person with diabetes the right to express a normal range of emotions. Even if you have diabetes, you can still get angry because you have something else to be angry about!

A Weapon of Manipulation

Diabetes provides a powerful pretext for emotional manipulation, up to the point of blackmail. Dietary requirements, obedience to rules (particularly regarding insulin), insulin reactions and diabetic comas, and physical disabilities are all sharp-edged weapons in the struggles between dependency and autonomy, freedom and control, resentment of confinement and fear of abandonment. They point in both directions. With food, for example (the dinner table is often a family battleground, even in the absence of diabetes): "I can't keep to my diet with all the rich foods you have around here" is met with "We can't eat what we want because we have to make so many allowances for you." Insulin routines and urine testing can be a prison of obligation and guilt for the family member with diabetes – who, to attack the prison walls, breaks the rules. A child gains attention by having an insulin reaction or developing keto-acidosis. A parent uses diabetes as a barrier to a growing child's independence by second-guessing every new step the child seeks to take: "Oh, no, *you* can't do that. You have diabetes."

An Obstacle to Romance

Dating and courtship can be strained by the reactions of the prospective partner and in-laws to diabetes. A parent or grandparent who has seen the effects of diabetes – or worse, knows of them only through hearsay – may advise (in the words of one man quoting his wife's father), "Steer clear of *that* – it's like buying a car when you know it's a lemon." A woman who experienced this stigma before her marriage describes some all-too-typical reactions:

> *Boyfriends' families don't like diabetic dates. One guy's mother said I wouldn't be able to have children. "Is that why you go out with her – because you're sorry for her?" she asked him. I'm pleased to note that I have outlived her.*
> *When I met my husband, he reacted with great equanimity. "Oh, my favorite aunt's diabetic," he said. But below the surface he was troubled, and it took us a few years before we decided to get married.*

The last part of this story is also typical. The revelation to a prospective mate that one has diabetes is a delicate matter. (Sometimes it is postponed as long as possible.) The mate may sidestep the issue out of loyalty or discomfort, but it needs to be worked through before marriage, as the man who provided the following account understood:

> By the time I met the woman I was to marry I could handle it pretty well. I had accepted the diabetes as a part of me, and if others didn't, it was their problem. With my wife it was a touchy subject at first. "Don't worry about it," she said. But I asked her to think about it – the fact that it would affect every part of our life together: eating, socializing, recreation, travel, sex. I asked her to visualize the possible long-term complications: my going blind, losing limbs, the children inheriting it. Finally she opened up to it. She read about it and asked me questions, and we went to the doctor together. Then she said she understood what the future might hold in store, and it was okay.

An Added Stress on Marriage

Diabetes (in either a spouse or child) adds stress to other factors threatening the stability of a marriage. With the family's energies focused on coping with diabetes, marital as well as parent-child problems are neglected until it is too late. Moreover, the diabetes itself is pressure against the point of an underlying weakness in a marriage, the point at which a tenuous equilibrium threatens to come unbalanced. Like poverty, diabetes in a spouse or child can be a catalyst of marital breakdown. People who might have muddled through in its absence end up divorced. They could not summon the mutual support to cope with such an ongoing crisis.

A Fear – and the Reality – of Abandonment

A major emotional issue in diabetes, as in all chronic illness, is fear of abandonment by loved ones. Whether this fear is justified depends on the strength of the relationship. When diabetes develops before marriage and the couple discusses it and reaches an understanding, the prospects are better than when diabetes develops after marriage, in a relationship not tested against this particular stress. In either case, though, disabling complications will test the relationship further. A counselor who leads diabetic retinopathy groups reports that three people in her groups have had engagements broken off by their fiancés. Our interviews are full of stories of spouses who withdrew emotionally and then physically: "My husband finally left because he couldn't handle it." "I broke off the marriage because I wasn't getting any real emotional support."

"Retinopathy makes a difficult thing more difficult," said a man who suffers from disabling vision loss. The "difficult thing" he referred to is intimacy. He was thinking of the time he went to a movie and asked his date to take his arm and lead him down the aisle because he could not see in the dark. But she went down the aisle without him, and he had to yell to her after the movie had started. At that moment he felt abandoned – a microcosm of larger betrayals. Abandonment is felt not only by intimate partners but also by blood relatives. Parents and siblings have been known to withdraw from the unfathomable challenges posed by a diabetic adolescent, particularly of the opposite sex. Family members are often far away, geographically or emotionally, when a crisis occurs in the life of a diabetic adult. A woman recalls suffering a series of hemorrhages: "The scary thing was not having a family to support me. My mother, sister, and brother were all living in different places and occupied with their own affairs. They couldn't or wouldn't set aside those things to come and help me, so I had to help myself."

For those with diabetes and its complications, the fear and reality of abandonment are an intensification of a universal dilemma. Intimate emotional loss is difficult to bear, even in the absence of loss of physical functioning. It isn't just people with retinopathy or amputated limbs – or even with diabetes – who are afraid to put themselves on the line and meet people again after rejection. Like anyone else in the same situation, they face two unhappy choices: accept loneliness as a permanent condition, or risk being abandoned again. And, like anyone else, they must make a value judgment and decide between the two.

A Resolution of Conflict and Mobilization of Mutual Support

Diabetes can strain a family relationship, but there are also positive effects. Diabetes may be the "last straw" that breaks up a failing marriage, but it has held together some couples who otherwise were headed for separation. Diabetes is a catalyst that brings issues to the surface, where they can be resolved to mutual benefit, particularly when parents, faced with the challenge of diabetes in a young child, set aside their differences for the child's sake. There is danger, though, in this otherwise inspiring scenario. The child, sensing that he or she needs to be ill to bring the parents together, may unconsciously exacerbate the illness whenever the parents seem to be drifting apart.

Diabetes, especially type 2, can serve as another kind of incentive: confronting previously unexamined emotional deadlocks that have over the years reinforced unhealthy living habits. Harry, a forty-five-year-old businessman, had never given much thought to why his repeated efforts to lose weight had been to no avail. But he could no longer evade the issue, once he developed type 2 diabetes and his doctor started asking pointed questions. It turned out that his wife, without realizing it, had been subtly sabotaging his attempts to diet by cooking rich meals and encouraging him to eat large portions. Overweight herself, and lacking confidence in the strength of their relationship, she feared a trimmer Harry might leave her for a more attractive woman. When diabetes raised the specter of losing Harry in a different and possibly final way, she was able to look more deeply at the implications of her behavior. She and Harry began to talk about their feelings for each other as they had not done in years, and they resolved to get thin together, rather than stay fat to stay together.

A Stimulus to Better Health Habits

Diabetes has another beneficial effect. It promotes greater health consciousness in the family. The challenge of preparing regular, healthful meals for a diabetic family member (without leading others, who are used to eating at odd times, to overeat) can be turned into an opportunity, if the family works at it together, to develop better eating habits. This experience of cooperation can in turn bring the family together emotionally. The wife of a man with non-insulin-dependent diabetes comments, "In creating a healthier dietary environment for Charlie I've come to have a whole different attitude toward food myself. I eat what I need to eat rather than what's immediately gratifying. As a result, I've lost a lot of weight and feel better, too." A shared period of exercise can be another way to benefit everyone individually and stimulate family closeness as well.

Family Responses

As much as diabetes affects family life, so (in less obvious but equally crucial ways) does family life affect the course of diabetes. For instance, parents who are absent, in conflict with each other, or ignorant or neglectful of their child's condition are not improving the chances that a child's diabetes will be well controlled (Hauser et al., 1990; Overstreet et al., 1995). On the other hand, it appears to be a two-way street. Family therapists increasingly look at family life as a "system" of interactions, far more complicated than parental influence alone, extending back to generations in which the roles now played by family members were established and expectations set for current generations. The family is characterized by mutual, rather than one-way, influence; for, while children initially learn from their parents how they are supposed to act, they set up their own demands and expectations that in turn lock their parents into implicitly prescribed patterns of behavior.

The following examples show how common patterns of family interaction play themselves out in response to diabetes and how they affect the course of the disease and its treatment.

Denial

If diabetes is too great a threat to a family's established way of functioning, the family may shut the illness out of its conscious-

Diabetes and the Family

ness as much as possible. With minimal attention from the family, treatment is likely to suffer. In addition, prevented from turning to the family, the member who has diabetes must rely on friends and professionals for emotional expression. In one reported case, the mother of an adolescent diabetic girl had not fully mourned the death of her own sister, who had been diabetic. As a result, unable to accept the implications of her daughter's diagnosis, she did not visit her in the hospital or become involved in her case. The daughter, who in turn could not mourn her own losses (of perfection, omnipotence, immortality), engaged in comparable forms of denial (Tarnow and Tomlinson, 1978).

The Sick Role

Some families divide themselves into givers and receivers of care. It is the role of some family members to express family tensions through physical illness, while others assume responsibility for their well-being. A child who takes on (that is, is assigned) the "sick role" lives out an exaggerated and prolonged version of childhood dependency, which serves the needs of overprotective parents as well as the child's own needs (as created by the family system). A child with diabetes may also be put in the sick role to enable other children in the family to appear strong and healthy by contrast (and perhaps to share the caretaking role with the parents).

Another common scenario for the sick role involves an adult man whose inattention to his diabetes (generally type 2) leaves his wife in charge of his diet. She then can either supervise him closely, which makes her appear an unpleasant nag, or leave him alone, risking guilt and recriminations for contributing to his irresponsibility. In one such family, a man in his seventies became increasingly childlike following the diagnosis of diabetes and the rapid appearance of complications affecting his vision, nerves, and circulation. Feeling that he had lost control of his body, he gave up control in other areas of his life as well, and relied on his wife to make his food and draw up his insulin. At the same time, he undercut her efforts by sneaking food like a child. His grown children joined him in this resistance: "Don't treat him that way," they told their mother. "He's an old man. Let him have what he wants." For her part, his wife felt responsible even if she was asleep when he got up during the night and ate ice cream. Needing to stay in control, but resenting the image of policewoman, she felt her closest family relationships compromised by the situation that had arisen around diabetes. Yet the situation had grown out of those very relationships.

The "Co-Diabetic" Role

The opposite number of the person in the "sick role" is the "co-diabetic" spouse, parent, or other relative – that is, a family member who takes on the life of the person with diabetes as his or her own. (The term is adapted from "co-alcoholic," which has a comparable meaning.) The person who assumes this role may be a mother whose constant worry about her child expresses a belief that the child's diabetes is punishment for her own unworthiness. It may be a father who, while his daughter is talking about her diabetes, breaks in and finishes the story himself. It may be a woman who marries her best friend's diabetic husband after the friend's death, stepping comfortably into the role of "nagging wife." It may be a person who chooses a diabetic mate to recreate the experience of living with a diabetic parent, or who takes on the role of the diabetic parent in a different guise. For example, a normally happy, outgoing man went through unpredictable mood swings in which he was susceptible to violent rages, which his family attributed to the effects of insulin. At those times his family "walked on eggshells" to avoid his wrath. One of his daughters married a man with a similar temperament; the other became alcoholic and put her children through the same insecurity and terror she had experienced with her father. As she put it, "My sister married Dad, and I grew up to be Dad."

The term "co-diabetic" describes a particular type of relationship. It is not a pejorative label automatically applied to anyone closely involved with a person who has diabetes. (We don't want to give you any problems you don't already have!) The term identifies one potentially dangerous way of living with diabetes. By looking at the examples given, you can see whether your family relationships fit the description and decide whether or not you want to do something about it.

The Diabetic Family

Diabetes is sometimes called a "family disease" because it is so closely tied in with family relationships and the shared experiences of everyday life. It has this character even when only one family member has it. At the extreme, there are families in which having diabetes is a normal state shared by several family members in two or three generations. In such a family (as in an example in Chapter 1), reaction to the diagnosis in one more family member may be matter-of-fact, and a child may gain greater acceptance by becoming like the parent and/or brothers and sisters who already have the disease.

Sibling Rivalry

Diabetes adds another dimension to the already complex relationships among brothers and sisters. Here are some common patterns to watch for in sibling relationships.

"Good" versus "bad" roles. If more than one child in the family has diabetes, they may differentiate themselves by taking on the roles of the "good diabetic" and the "bad diabetic." This form of rivalry locks the "good" and "bad" siblings into patterns of behavior that are not necessarily conducive – and often detrimental – to their well-being.

Competition for attention. While a diabetic child may envy a brother or sister who is free to eat, the non-diabetic sibling has something to envy, too – namely, the constant attention given the diabetic sibling. The child with diabetes is "special." This has its compensations, especially from the point of view of another child who may feel a relative lack of nurturance, while not feeling the pain that comes with having diabetes.

Extreme fear. Underneath the nonchalance of the child who does not have diabetes there may lie terror at the prospect of suffering that fate. In one family a brother of the child with diabetes announced that he was coming "under protest" to family therapy sessions, where he would dribble a basketball while family members shared their feelings. It took several sessions for him to admit to being terrified that he, too, might develop diabetes.

Psychosomatic Reactions

In several of our interviews, a child or adolescent developed diabetes shortly after the parents separated or remarried. This might be coincidental; that is, some children might experience onset at such times simply by chance, but the timing would appear significant to their families. However, it seems likely that family stress can precipitate onset when the disease process is underway.

Once diabetes has developed, the quality of family life appears clearly related to blood sugar control and the frequency of episodes of keto-acidosis and insulin reactions (Jacobson et al., 1994). In particular, numerous studies draw a connection between a mother's style of childrearing and the level of metabolic control observed in her diabetic child. These studies identify four types of maternal attitudes that have a generally harmful effect on diabetes control. These are (with illustrative quotations from our interviews):

- overprotective; overanxious ("They wove a cocoon around me, their poor little boy with diabetes.")

- overindulgent; overpermissive ("I just did what the rest of the family did – when I ate too much, I took more insulin to compensate.")

- perfectionist; controlling ("My mother was like the local pediatrician; she regulated my insulin with four tests a day, and anything less than a negative test drove her crazy.")

- indifferent; rejecting ("My mother had babies, not children.")

The observed effects of these styles of parenting have been summarized as follows:

> *Parental indifference had the most serious effect on the diabetic child, leading to depression and the poorest levels of metabolic control. Perfectionistic, overcontrolling mothers had children with excellent or satisfactory regulation of the disease but who were rebellious. Both overindulgent and overprotective maternal styles led to maladjusted children with low levels of adherence. Finally, mothers described as tolerant, consistent, and flexible were reported to have children who were both well adjusted and in satisfactory metabolic control.* (Anderson and Auslander, 1980)

If a man develops type 1 diabetes soon after his wife leaves him, we cannot speak with any assurance about the connection between the two events. But suppose he ends up in the emergency room with keto-acidosis because, having already developed diabetes, he stopped taking his insulin when his marriage broke up. There we can draw a clear connection. Similarly, if he develops type 2 diabetes (not previously diagnosed) because he gained forty pounds after the separation, a behavioral link is evident. The same is true for the parent-child relationship. The effects of family stress on metabolic control operate at both the behavioral and psychosomatic levels. If parental nurturance, training, and supervision are not all they could be, the child (whether out of ignorance or defiance) will not take the most effective steps toward blood sugar control. In addition, researchers have identified some children whose emotional state has had a direct effect on their diabetic metabolism (Cox and Gonder-Frederick, 1992; Surwit and Schneider, 1993). Stressful events in the household can throw these children's blood sugar levels out of control, even if the children stick to their treatment regimens.

What is most disturbing, some children suffer metabolic disturbances without deviating from their treatment routines. Moreover, they do so, in effect, "on cue." That is, their particular version of the "sick role" involves more than invalidism or misbehavior. It actually calls for an attack of keto-acidosis to be triggered when family conflict rises to such a level that a dramatic event is needed to divert energy from the conflict and bring the family together again. Family therapist Salvador Minuchin and his colleagues have identified four characteristics of the family environment that (together with the child's physiological vulnerability) put a child at risk for this dangerous pattern of psychosomatic reactions:

1. *Enmeshment* – a situation in which family members are so deeply involved with, and highly responsive to, one another that individual identities and roles become unclear.
2. *Overprotectiveness* – a tacit agreement by which all family members protect one another from conflict and pain, extending beyond illness to normal rough spots in life.
3. *Rigidity* – a shared commitment to maintaining the status quo.
4. *Lack of conflict resolution* – an ingrained habit of avoiding rather than explicitly negotiating differences.

When these arrangements are stretched to the limit, the "safety valve" represented by the child's blood sugar is "released," and the family closes ranks around the medical emergency. Equilibrium is thus restored (Minuchin et al., 1975). Although the validity of the Minuchin model has been questioned (Coyne and Anderson, 1988; 1989), it may still provide a useful framework for understanding particular cases.

In a fascinating case study, Minuchin and Barcai (1969) describe how family therapy worked in the case of Julie, age twelve, who experienced repeated, potentially life-threatening bouts of keto-acidosis. Her physicians had given up their attempts to control her condition medically and referred her to family therapists, who redefined the problem as a family rather than a medical one. Observing the way family members consistently played to each other's roles to keep the existing family structure intact, the therapists gave the family members instructions designed to violate the rules and break down the system. They thus precipitated a crisis during which (as expected) Julie had even more medical emergencies than usual. In the long run, however, the frequency of her hospitalizations dropped drastically. Meanwhile, her brothers and sisters began to get into trouble in other ways as each in turn took over the role of "weak" family member from Julie. Family therapy continued to focus on each individual's problems in the context of the overall family system.

In a more recent case, fourteen-year-old Chris had been hospitalized sixty-six times in five years despite conscientious care by his parents. It appeared that he could not live much longer – at least outside the hospital. Family therapy with his parents and sister revealed that Chris was caught between his father's wish that he be more independent and his mother's need to shelter him. Initially Chris resisted therapy. "I didn't want things to change," he said. "I liked the old way better when everyone would baby me." The therapist brought about a crisis by prodding the father to get tough with Chris and the mother to support her husband instead of defending her son. This emotional catharsis led to Chris's being able to grow up and stay in good diabetic control while his family became free to have a normal life together. "The biggest difference is that our family no longer has diabetes," his father reflected. "Chris has it and we are no longer his conscience" (Hochman, 1984).

Positive Models

What about all the families in which a person with diabetes is supported in achieving the best possible state of health? No generalizations can encompass all the ways in which a family can nurture; different styles work for different families. But researchers and clinicians have observed some general qualities that many effective families share. Parental self-esteem is crucial in determining how well a child will function with diabetes (Grey et al., 1980). More generally, families of children with well-controlled diabetes have been found to have the following characteristics:

1. *Family life is stable.*
2. *Family members enjoy each other's company.*
3. *Boundaries between the generations are intact, with each generation having its own distinct identity and place in the family.*

4. *Attitudes toward diabetes care are realistic and responsible.*
5. *If the loss of a parent has occurred, it is made up for by the ego-strength of the remaining parent.* (Koski et al., 1976)

Good parent-child communication is essential, both about feelings (Jacobson et al., 1994) and about shared responsibilities for diabetes care (Anderson et al., 1990).

Here is one description of a supportive family environment:

> *Ideally, the stable, harmonious family . . . provides the diabetic [child] with a supportive, consistent environment, promoting open discussion about the illness, its management, its causes and uncertain future course, its negative influence on the family's daily life and plans, etc. – all the time showing respect for where the child or adolescent is – in terms of emotional and cognitive-intellectual development.* (Mattsson, 1979)

A large order, perhaps, but one that some families do approximate. When six-year-old Larry developed diabetes, his parents resolved to allow him as normal a life as possible without denying or neglecting the illness. They discussed diabetes matter-of-factly with Larry and his two sisters, making clear that it was not something to be ashamed of but did require special attention and care. Family meals were planned with Larry's needs in mind, on the understanding that the balanced diet required for diabetes would be good for everyone. At the same time, no restrictions were placed on what foods other family members could have in the house or eat on the outside. Larry's parents arranged to have a responsible baby-sitter come in one night a week so that they could regularly have some time "off to themselves." They did not want to feel as if their own lives had been engulfed by Larry's diabetes. They attended to Larry's blood sugar regulation with close but not harsh supervision, explaining the importance of good control but letting Larry know they understood his personal needs as well. As his mother explained, "We didn't want to come down so hard on him that he'd need to 'cheat' on the outside or rebel in some other harmful way."

In this tolerant, relaxed atmosphere, Larry learned that he could be open and honest about having diabetes, and conflicts with his sisters were minimized. In his teens Larry gradually took over his own diabetes management and remained in good control. He excelled in school and was recognized as a leader in activities where he could use his considerable skill in dealing with people, a skill he had picked up at home. With the sound preparation for life his parents had given him, Larry faced the future with confidence.

Guidelines for Families

The following recommendations should prove useful in negotiating the delicate interplay between family life and diabetes care:

Don't attribute everything that goes on in the family to diabetes. A family is made up of people, and having diabetes is only one small part of what a person is. Keep the diabetes in perspective by remembering that people do what they do for reasons that are almost always prior to and independent of the appearance of diabetes in the family.

Know how and when to confront. If you observe a family member acting self-destructively with regard to diabetes, or being destructive to or overly dependent on anyone else (a dependency you feel is a burden), ask yourself the following questions before you confront him or her:

1. Has the communication been solicited rather than imposed? Have you asked permission to make it?
2. Is the person in any shape to hear it, or is the person too fragile?
3. Has he or she heard it before? how many times?
4. Is the communication descriptive rather than evaluative? Is it about what you see or what you think should be? How much of your own bias enters into it?
5. Is it something the person can do something about? Are the issues negotiable, or are you asking the person to be what he or she is not?

6. Is this the right time for it?
7. Is it worth the hassle – to both of you – to say this? Can the relationship bear the strain and conflict that may result?

Variations on these questions apply whether you are considering ending a relationship or wondering how best to advise a loved one. In the former case, what you then have to say is very personal. In the latter, you will want to challenge, contradict, and question in a nonpunitive way. Here is one formula for doing so:

"What do you want?"
"What are you doing?"
"Will doing what you're doing help you get what you want?"

Don't be fatalistic. Diabetes does not necessarily bring about a deterioration in an individual's emotional health or in the quality of a family's life. On the contrary, researchers have found inspiring evidence of resilience in people who have faced the challenges of diabetes. In one study, mothers' anxiety and depression increased after a child was diagnosed with diabetes, but returned to normal levels in the years that followed (Kovacs et al., 1990a). Equally reassuring for parents is the finding that young adults diagnosed ten years earlier with diabetes appeared to be as well adjusted psychologically as young adults who did not have a chronic illness (Jacobson et al., 1997).

Try family therapy as needed. If your family could benefit from a fresh perspective and guidance in coping more effectively with diabetes, various forms of family therapy may prove helpful (Rubin and Peyrot, 1992; Satin et al., 1989). For example, one innovative approach succeeded in improving children's blood sugar control by reducing the stress on their parents (Guthrie et al., 1990).

Live with, not for, diabetes. This tip is as important for families as it is for individuals. A family's life, like an individual's, need not center around diabetes. You must live with diabetes, but you don't have to live for it.

Diabetes and the Family

For Further Reading

American Diabetes Association. *Diabetes in the Family* (rev. ed.). Alexandria, VA: American Diabetes Association, 1987.

Hochman, G. Does your family make you sick . . . or well? *American Health* 3(7) (1984):74–87.

Rubin, R.R., Biermann, J., and Toohey, B. *Psyching Out Diabetes: A Positive Approach to Your Negative Emotions.* Los Angeles: Lowell House, 1992.

For Parents

For Mary and Paul Kozlowski, it was as if their lives had been turned inside out. They had told Amy they would go to Burger King after the doctor looked at her to see why she was wetting her bed so much. Instead, they went straight to the hospital. Amy, three years old, remained there for two weeks to get her diabetes under control. "It ripped my heart right out," Mary recalled. "I didn't think I'd make it through the first week. I'd look at this tiny kid with an IV stuck in her, and I'd think, 'This is a dream; it isn't really happening. We'll go home and it'll all be over.'"

At the beginning there was a lot of confusion and feelings of fear, anger, and guilt that would not entirely disappear. But the Kozlowskis did learn to cope, even during the first year when Amy hardly understood what had happened to her. In all the decisions and dilemmas they faced that year, what may have helped most was simply keeping in mind that, as Paul put it, "With or without the diabetes, she's still a little girl."

Diabetes, such a massive presence in an individual's and a family's life, is often blamed for any problem that comes up, as if people who don't have diabetes don't run into the same problems. Sometimes it appears that people who don't have diabetes never argue with their spouse or boss, never end up divorced or out of a job. In the same vein, parents of children with diabetes imagine that children who don't have diabetes never exceed their limits, never feel deprived, never fight with their brothers and sisters, never come home crying, never stalk angrily out the door. In the sugarplum world of families who don't have diabetes, surely parents and children don't fight; with no rules and restrictions, there's nothing to fight about. Such lucky children don't have many rules and restrictions to contend with, and they accept the ones they have. Parents of healthy children don't worry when they begin to venture out into the world and make mistakes, because they are not life-or-death mistakes. And so the fantasy goes.

If your child has diabetes, bear in mind that what appears to be a diabetic problem is usually a child development issue as well, one that would come up in one form or another, even in the absence of diabetes. Diabetes may intensify, diminish, or alter these "growing pains." It may furnish a convenient excuse or focus for their expression. But rarely does it create them. It does, however, raise the ante. Most conflicts between parents and children do not have life-or-death consequences (at least until the child reaches driving age). But when a child's tantrum, or an adolescent's rebellion, undermines good diabetes management, then there is indeed a great deal at stake. This added, impersonal "punishment" for doing what anyone else might do is part of the emotional burden of diabetes both for the child and for the parents.

Consider how a child extends the boundaries of his or her world by exploring the neighborhood – and beyond – on a bicycle. Children sometimes disagree with their parents when it comes to setting boundaries for bike riding at a particular age, and they also have been known to venture outside these boundaries. In the case of a diabetic child, however, there is an added concern: "What if you have a reaction?" When questions like these come up, take a look at both sides of the issue and, when necessary, disentangle them. Step back and ask yourselves, "How much of this is about diabetes, and how much is it about childhood (or adolescence)?" With experience (some of which will be tense and frustrating), you can develop a good intuitive grasp of your child's physical, emotional, and developmental needs.

Battlegrounds

The battle that parents and child together fight for good diabetes control within a fulfilling life is predictably waged over those areas of daily life in which the diabetic child feels least "normal," most set apart from other children. Food, insulin, urine and blood sugar testing, and restricted activity are areas of tension in the life of a child with diabetes, and they can also provoke tension between child and parents.

Food

Food has many meanings for children, especially in our society where sweet foods are associated with pleasure and used as a reward for good behavior. Ironically, to be a "good diabetic," a child must do without what previously was proof of being "good." No wonder diet is more of a problem than insulin! And, if it is painful for the child to be denied certain foods, it is also painful for parents to withhold them. It removes an important outlet for expressing love and providing nurturance.

Insulin

Most children get used to the inconvenience and pain of insulin injections more readily than parents might expect. But giving an injection still has overtones of assault, especially for a very young child, and the child's pain is shared by the parents who see themselves as inflicting it. At the same time, insulin is a gift of life. Parents innocently fail to realize that a child old enough to understand what insulin is can appreciate the love with which it is given. In this way, parents can feel they are nurturing, their child, in a deep sense, when they give insulin.

Testing

If an insulin injection can be experienced as an assault, so can a painful needle prick in the finger. Urine testing, meanwhile, goes against the parental admonition that it is strictly taboo to play with what you secrete and excrete. (Thank goodness diabetes doesn't call for daily stool samples!) Even when testing is not physically painful, it can be felt as an intrusion into the child's private world. "Did you check your urine?" sounds like "Did you brush your teeth?" "Did you roll up all the car windows?" "Show me your homework!" – another unwelcome inquisition, repeated perhaps four times a day. For this reason, the growing medical evidence that frequent testing does improve one's long-range prospects for health may create difficult choices for parents who are sensitive to their child's need for privacy.

Restrictions on Activity

This is an area where diabetes may further strain the already raw nerves of parent-child relations; for example, the boundaries for bicycle riding. Should an eight-year-old go trick-or-treating alone? Will the kid down the street be a bad influence? When can a child (or adolescent) be trusted to stay overnight with a friend? Is it worth the time and risk of injury to try out for the football team? Will a driver's license put a sixteen-year-old beyond the reach of parental guidance? Is the teenager out late at night experimenting with drugs and sex? What about that youth hosteling expedition through Europe? Questions like these come up in any family with growing children. Sometimes the child's diabetes is overemphasized when actually it is incidental to adolescent rites of passage. On the other hand, diabetes sometimes adds to the frustration of growing up by posing real obstacles to a child's participation in activities that other children take for granted.

Natural Reactions: Anxiety and Guilt

Parents would worry about their children even if there were no such thing as diabetes. But the diagnosis of diabetes, and with it the realization of an immediate, lifelong need to bring a fluctuating blood sugar level under control, raises anxiety to a fever pitch. You may recognize your own initial feelings in Mary Kozlowski's story at the beginning of this chapter, or in a thirty-year-old man's recollection of his parents' "subtle, harried frenzy" when they first took him to the hospital twenty years earlier. Because of this normal parental anxiety, doctors and nurses learn not to overwhelm either the parents or the child with information right away. For parents, it may be wise not to try to learn everything at once. Once your child's blood sugar is under control for the time being, it makes sense just to live with the disease for a while, to get accustomed to it, to do what is necessary from day to day, and to ask questions as they occur to you and as you are able to fit the answers into the child's daily routine. Remember, anxiety is contagious. Children take their cues from their parents. Anxiety is a normal reaction for both parents and child, but it can become excessive. For example, a physician insisted that his son urinate into a cup in his presence so that he could be sure that the right urine was being tested. Although this father's worry was understandable, his way of expressing it was inappropriate – not likely to help the child's adjustment to diabetes.

A second near-universal reaction is guilt. Guilt can have more damaging effects than anxiety precisely because it is more often hidden. First you feel guilty, then you feel guilty about feeling guilty, so you keep it to yourself. Guilt is indeed an uncomfortable feeling, and the things that you feel guilty about can be difficult to talk about. That is why it is so important to see how common, how natural, it is for parents of diabetic children to doubt, question, and blame themselves, even though they are not to blame. This is one time when you really are – as the saying goes – not alone.

Guilt about Heredity

Because diabetes has a hereditary component, a parent who has diabetes, or who has a family history of diabetes, may feel guilty about having "given" diabetes to his or her child. Occasionally the guilt is made worse when he or she is blamed by the other parent for having "passed on" the disease. Although this seems like a heartless thing to do, it can be understood as an expression of grief over the child's illness, and it needs to be resolved by both parents together through counseling. Feelings of guilt can also be reinforced by well-intentioned medical personnel, as Joan Hoover relates:

A teaching nurse I know has the parents of a newly diagnosed diabetic child diagram a family tree and identify the diabetic members. This is so they can better understand how their child came to be diabetic. Now, aside from being bad science, what kind of totally nonproductive guilt trip is that to lay on a family? (Hoover, 1979)

What Hoover means by "bad science" is that heredity is only one of many causes of diabetes, and the nature and extent of its causal role are not well understood. The transmission of diabetes from parent to child is far from automatic. Diabetes often skips generations and sometimes affects only one child in a large family. According to current estimates, a child with only one type 1 diabetic parent has a 2- to 10-percent chance of developing type 1 diabetes. If both parents have the disease, the risk is thought to range from 30 to 50 percent. Even then, by one estimate, the probability that diabetes will show up before the age of twenty is only 12 to 15 percent.

With type 2 diabetes, the hereditary link is stronger. The probability that the identical twin of a person with type 2 diabetes will also be diabetic is at least 95 percent. It is only 30 to 50 percent for type 1. Even so, parental guilt is not as likely to be an issue with type 2 as with type 1. In the first place, type 2 diabetes develops undramatically and seldom occurs in childhood, although it is showing up increasingly in obese, sedentary adolescents (Pinhas-Hamiel and Zeitler, 1997). If you have type 2 diabetes, chances are you had children before you knew you had it (although you may have known that it was in your family). And your children most likely will have twenty or thirty years' "notice," during which time they can prevent – or retard – the onset of the disease through weight control and regular exercise. Finally, no hereditary link *between* the two types of diabetes has been established.

Diabetes does run in families, but it runs a mysterious course. What with the irregularities of transmission and age at onset, it would be impossible to eliminate diabetes from the human gene pool, even if all those known to have diabetes had no children. The parents of a diabetic child deserve compassion and support, not censure, most of all from themselves. In their anguish over their child's suffering they may worry that they have wronged the child. But was it wrong to give life to this child they now love?

It is only prudent for those who have diabetes in their family backgrounds to discuss the genetic implications with their prospective spouses and, where further information is needed, or where some uneasiness or disagreement remains, to clarify the issues through genetic counseling. (This is especially useful when there is diabetes on both sides of the family-to-be.) But the transmission of a genetic susceptibility to disease is not the same as deliberate or negligent wrongdoing.

Still, to say that you *need* not feel guilty is not the same as saying that you *will* not feel guilty. Helpful as it is to put things in perspective, guilt can be a pretty persistent feeling. When guilt gets in the way of doing what is best for your child and for yourself, it makes sense to talk things over with a trained counselor.

Other "Triggers" of Guilt

You don't need to have diabetes yourself or in your family to feel pangs of guilt toward a diabetic child. The deprivations and assaults that diabetes care entails are reason enough. Who can feel easy about denying a child desserts and hurting the child with needles, even when it is all done with the best of motives? Worst of all is when the child is too young to understand the reasons for the sacrifice and pain. Three-year-old Amy Kozlowski used to say to her parents, "Stop giving me the shot, and I won't have diabetes anymore." This fantasy that the parent is "giving" the child diabetes with the insulin injection is common in very young children, but the parent at whom it is directed suffers alone. Two weeks after her initial hospitalization, when they were going back to the hospital for further consultation, Amy asked her mother, "Are we going there to give back the diabetes, or are they going to give me more of it?" To Mary Kozlowski, "It was devastating that she would think that somehow I had contributed to it." Fortunately, with the help of some patient explanation, Amy learned to distinguish between the illness and its treatment. While she did not understand how insulin worked, she could grasp that it was "medicine."

Sometimes parents feel guilty for what seems to be "no reason at all." It was Paul Kozlowski who had diabetes in his family, but it was Mary who blamed herself. "If it had been *my* father who had it," she reflected, "I imagine I would have been overwhelmed with guilt. As it is, I say to myself, maybe I smoked too many cigarettes when I was pregnant, maybe I did something stupid in my teens." Here the idea of being punished for past sins takes the form of a biological explanation, but Mary also experienced it in almost purely religious terms:

> *It really hits me sometimes at night when Amy looks so peaceful lying there asleep. I wonder what I did, that this should be visited upon her. It seems to me now that I had it made before, only I was ungrateful, and then this happened.*

Mary knew only too well that this way of thinking is irrational. When she got to brooding too long and deeply, she knew enough to stop and remind herself, "This happened to Amy, not to me." But no amount of good sense can make one immune to recurrent feelings of guilt. Parental responsibility is a deeply rooted instinct that asserts itself regardless of reason and logic. In one poignant case, a woman in her twenties suffering from advanced diabetic retinopathy underwent laser surgery in an effort to reverse or retard her loss of vision. In her case the operation was not successful; it left her with a further loss of vision, which probably would have occurred anyway during the next few years. Her father, who lived in another part of the country, continued to feel guilty. "I was right there, and I didn't stop them from doing it" – this despite the fact that his daughter was an adult who had chosen to take a reasonable risk after consultation with several physicians as well as her family.

Perhaps the most important thing you can do to keep parental guilt from getting out of hand is to understand it as a normal reaction. Anyone in your position would have it to some degree. Other parents of children with diabetes will also tell you that it is normal for guilt to lessen as time passes. It may never completely go away; it may occasionally be intense when something comes up that reminds you of past events and emotions; but if you continue to dwell on it, you risk doing yourself and your child real harm. An unremitting sense of guilt can lead to helplessness, depression, overcompensation, martyrdom, and less-than-optimal decision making. It can trap you in the thankless, self-sacrificing "co-diabetic" role discussed in the previous chapter.

If you are having difficulty getting past the kind of overwhelming guilt that Mary Kozlowski experienced, share your concerns with someone you feel you can trust to respond sensitively. It may be someone in your family, the child's physician, or perhaps a sympathetic nurse. Ideally, all medical personnel who work with juvenile diabetes should be sensitive to the emotional toll this disease exacts on parents and trained to help parents bring uncomfortable feelings out into the open. If not, you still have other options. Check the web sites and organizations listed at the back of this book. Contact other parents who have been through the same thing; see if there is a parents' support group in your area, or start one. If that doesn't work, seek professional help. Perhaps all you need is a few sessions to air your feelings and get a different perspective on them.

An Everyday "Crisis"

A parent's judgment can be thrown off course by anxiety and guilt; yet responsible decision making can proceed in the midst of these emotions. The following paragraphs recount a typical dilemma faced by the parents of a diabetic child.

Four-year-old Amy is out playing with her friends. When bells ring to announce the arrival of the ice cream truck, the other kids run to their parents for money. Amy wants ice cream, too, but she is not exercising hard enough to work off the extra sugar. What should her parents do?

Here are three different ways in which a family might handle the situation:

Mr. and Mrs. Jones, feeling guilty about all the times they have to say no to Amy, let her have the ice cream. That night Amy is ill. Mrs. Jones, agitated and unsure of herself, blames the child. "You see?" she admonishes her. "You were the one who wanted the ice cream. You were the one who ate it."

Mr. and Mrs. Smith explain to Amy that this is not a good time for her to eat ice cream. "But you *can* have a piece of fruit," they suggest, "and you can have ice cream tomorrow before you swim." Or else they may give her a sugar-free ice cream bar from their own freezer.

Mr. and Mrs. Kozlowski, recognizing how important it is for Amy to identify with and be accepted by her peers, let her buy the ice cream, but let her eat only part of it. They experiment with the size of the portion to see what she can tolerate without getting sick. They are willing to risk an occasional hyperglycemic episode for the sake of her emotional well-being and social adjustment. They are concerned, moreover, that, if they never let her have ice cream or cake with her friends, she might eat these things behind their back. As it is, Amy is learning her own limits and the consequences of exceeding them.

It is clear that Mr. and Mrs. Jones's response does not work as well as the other two. The Joneses let guilt and anxiety govern their actions, and both they and the child end up unhappy. In this scenario Amy gets the ice cream, but she also gets her parents' guilt projected onto her.

Parents like the Joneses can take heart in seeing that there is more than one way to do it "right." The Smiths and Kozlowskis, in their different ways, both take responsibility for making parental decisions. The Smiths exert strong but nurturant authority; the Kozlowskis allow more flexibility. The Smiths place primary emphasis on dietary regulation and blood sugar control; the Kozlowskis are also concerned with Amy's relationships with other children. Choosing between the two approaches involves a complex value judgment, an assessment of costs and benefits that takes into consideration the child's present as well as future well-being.

It is valuable for any four-year-old to learn to delay gratification, as Amy Smith is learning, especially with the help of a careful explanation showing that the restrictions are not arbitrary. On the other hand, most four-year-olds don't have to learn that lesson when the ice cream truck comes. Amy Kozlowski is getting a lesson in self-regulation within carefully set limits. For her the question is whether she is ready for this responsibility, and what the long-term physical effects of a less restrictive diet will be. Whether her parents or the Smiths are "right" depends on the particular child and the particular situation; it may depend as well on medical knowledge that we don't yet possess.

The Issues at Stake

Now we can take a look at the larger issues illustrated by our vignette. What guidelines should parents keep in mind for balancing healthy child development and the care of childhood diabetes? What are some of the different guises in which the same underlying questions can arise? What are the common pitfalls for parent and child?

Independence versus Tender Loving Care

A child with diabetes requires a great deal of special care. Yet this same child must be trained for a lifetime of self-management. Both needs must be met without going overboard in either direction. For parents, the danger is in being too nurturant on the one hand or too demanding on the other.

Overprotectiveness. Diabetes gives parents another reason (as if they didn't have enough already) to smother their children with love and concern. Parents, in an effort to make up for the child's metabolic vulnerability and/or whatever deficiencies they ascribe to themselves, may engage in well-intentioned overregulation that does more harm than good: for example, shielding the child from normal activity – playing, socializing, physical exertion. Parents of diabetic children are not the only ones to feel this impulse or to act on it. But diabetes does give added cause for worry about what might happen when the child is not under direct parental observation and control.

We see overprotectiveness in diabetes management as well. "More is better" is not appropriate for insulin dosages. Overdosing a child's insulin in an attempt to achieve consistently "good" test results can have deleterious medical consequences ranging from hypoglycemia to acquired insensitivity to insulin.

Overtesting is a more subtle issue than overtreatment. The Diabetes Control and Complications Trial (DCCT) demonstrated that the more you test, the more you learn, and the better you can regulate your child's blood sugar. The better control you achieve, the better your child's chances of avoiding damaging complications later in life (Brink and Moltz, 1997). Even so, there is still a place for commonsense in deciding when and how to test. By all means, test frequently at the outset, as well as when your child eats something unusual or at an odd time of day. Keep track of the effects of growth. But be conscious as well of the intrusion and weigh this cost against the benefits of testing. How does your child feel about blood and urine tests? Have you fully explained the reasons for testing often? As your child's condition stabilizes, try to sense when testing may have diminishing returns. Perhaps most important, avoid a judgmental attitude. The purpose of testing is, through feedback, to improve blood sugar control. It is not a means of checking up on a child with all the unpleasantness and combativeness that that entails.

For the first few weeks after Amy Kozlowski came home from the hospital, her mother and father hovered over her, watching for the slightest pretext to test her blood sugar. It took months for them to stop taking more tests each day than their physician recommended. They were worried about Amy, of course, but they were also worried about being "good" parents. In other words, all that testing was serving their needs as well as (perhaps more than) Amy's. As Mary put it, "My biggest fear, ten times a day, is 'Is she all right? Will she have a reaction when I'm not there? Or will she have one when I'm the only one there, and I won't be able to handle it?'" She and Paul needed to learn from experience that it takes time for blood sugar to rise to a dangerous level. They needed to make mistakes and see that these were not fatal. In retrospect, they could laugh at mishaps like this:

> *A couple of weeks after we brought Amy home from the hospital we were sitting watching TV, and we noticed that she was sweating. Right away we drew up some glucagon (which has to be used immediately; it can't be put back). We were about to inject it when we thought, "What the hell – we'd better do a test first." She tested at 200; there was nothing wrong with her. We had wasted $15 worth of glucagon when she was just hot and sweaty. The kid was fine, and here we were, two nervous wrecks.*

When you find yourself frequently rushing to test or treat, ask, "What are we learning or accomplishing by this? Whose needs are being served? Is it for the child or for us?"

Overcompensation. Parents may respond to anxiety and guilt by going to the other extreme – i.e., demanding too much independence too quickly. Exercise is often a battleground for parentally imposed overachievement. An anxious parent reacts to a child's "bad" test results by taking the whole family out for a run around the block, or pushes and prods the child to use an exercise bicycle. Most children relish physical activity. But when exercise is made the object of overenthusiastic parental coaching, a child may come to think of it as though it were . . . well, like playing the piano when you want to play ball. A struggle for control ensues. The parent's concern is pitted against the natural contrariness of the child. Lost in the struggle is the exercise the child really does need. If you find yourself locked in this confrontational posture, break loose from the clinch. Better to use words like these: "It's important that you exercise for the sake of your health. This matters to me because I love you, but I know you're the one who's living with it."

Parents sometimes push children to administer their own insulin (and even to regulate their own dosage) too soon. This too is over-compensation. Children must eventually learn to take their own injections, so parents naturally are reassured to see a child master this skill as quickly as possible. Parental pride is also involved. Ask yourself again, "Whose needs are being served? Who needs to have the child be self-sufficient with insulin right away?" Parents have a legitimate concern that their child develop independence and responsibility, but it is a fallacy to think that a child who doesn't inject his or her own insulin at the age of ten will not do it at twenty. Children do grow up, in this way as in others. As a matter of fact, in the experience of some clinicians, it is the children who do inject themselves at an early age who are more likely to have difficulties later on.

Insulin is a matter of life and death. For the young child who needs it, it is part of the food, clothing, shelter, and protection from harm for which the child looks to his or her parents. These parental gifts reassure the child and nourish an emotional security out of which the adolescent shapes an independent identity. Thus, while a child of any age can practice giving injections, a child does not need to do it for real until he or she has indicated a clear readiness for the task. When is a child ready? At four, Amy Kozlowski participates by rating each shot: "That's pretty good," or "That one hurt." In another year or two she will be able to push down the plunger. At eleven or twelve she should be able to draw up the insulin and inject herself, and when she is fifteen or sixteen she can begin to regulate her own dosage. These ages are illustrative only; the pace depends on the individual child. Children eager to assume responsibility earlier can be encouraged to do so. The important thing to remember is that the child learns self-care in stages and will still require supervision at each stage (Anderson and Laffel, 1997). After all, children do not learn all at once to choose their own clothing, and parents do not entrust them with unlimited funds for this purpose. Parents should be prepared to hear an adolescent, weaned from parental insulin injections, say, "I don't want to do my own shot tonight; please do it for me." The child is seeking reassurance that the parents' supportive presence is still there when needed.

Life and growth will create the incentives for the child to outgrow dependency. At the same time, the child's evolving social environment can provide peer support for – as well as challenges to – responsible diabetes care (La Greca, 1991; La Greca et al., 1995). For many children, a key passage comes around the ages of eleven to thirteen when they begin to want to stay overnight with friends. Now they have a reason to be medically self-sufficient. Parents can welcome this development with the understanding that complete self-sufficiency will not be achieved all at once. One twelve-year-old girl called her mother from a friend's house, where she was to spend the night, and announced, "I forgot my insulin." Her mother calmly replied, "Well, Jennifer, what do you think we should do?" Instead of reproaching her daughter, she asked her to share responsibility for solving the problem. Jennifer suggested, "Maybe I can get a ride home to pick it up." "Yes," said her mother, "or else Daddy can bring it over." There was no confrontation, no harsh judgment, no assault on Jennifer's self-esteem. The focus was on correcting the mistake – a mistake, the mother realized, any adult might have made.

Finding the right balance of autonomy and guidance for a particular child can be a delicate matter. One mother had to be counseled to get beyond the anxiety that kept her from realizing that her recently diagnosed seventeen-year-old son was intelligent and mature enough to take care of himself. On the other hand, a young man of nineteen, who had taken an independent stance since onset at age twelve, reflected wistfully, "I wish I hadn't had my parents back off so much, which they did in other areas besides the diabetes." Having learned to take responsibility at an early age, he felt responsible for his parents' behavior as well as his own.

Limit-Testing and Normal Development

All children need limits and at the same time are frustrated by them. Children with diabetes have more than the usual number of limits to contend with. Diabetes brings parents and children into close contact and sets up additional areas for conflict over issues of control. However, the wise parent understands such conflicts as variations on a theme with which any parent is familiar.

Limit-testing in the diabetic child can be fueled by a sense of entitlement based on deprivation: "Since I can't have what other kids have, I can take something else." Where does the child pick up this reasoning? In part, it seems, from the parents' guilt and a certain permissiveness that this engenders. The tug-of-war begins very early in the course of the illness and very early in life, as Paul Kozlowski can attest:

> It didn't take Amy a week to learn that she could get away with things. One day in the hospital she was lying in bed, perfectly fine, when suddenly she rolled over on her stomach and didn't move. "Ice cream – I feel funny," she moaned, because she remembered that they had given her ice cream once before when her sugar was low. We were really scared until we saw her peeking with one eye and smiling. Now when she says she won't do something (like pick up her toys) because she doesn't feel good, I'll pull out the glucometer, test her on the spot, and punish her if she's faking.
>
> For a while she drove me up the wall whenever she held us up by dawdling over a meal. Since she couldn't be allowed to miss a meal, she could make us late whenever she wanted. Now we make like we're going out the door and tell her, "If you're not finished eating when we get out to the car, you'll have to stay here alone all day." Then she gobbles it down, and we're on our way. Sometimes she's actually said, "I won't eat my lunch if you don't let me have. . . ." So we say, "Okay, so you won't eat lunch." Eventually it will be all her responsibility, and even now it's her choice whether or not to eat.

It was incidents like these that led Paul to remark, "With or without the diabetes, she's still a little girl." As they have gained experience, he and Mary have responded to Amy's acting out with firm discipline and a refusal to be manipulated, just as they would if she did not have diabetes. At first sight it may seem like nuclear brinksmanship to call a diabetic child's bluff about missing a meal. But of all the children who have threatened to hold their breath to the point of losing consciousness, how many have actually done so?

As your child grows, different issues arise during normal development, with an increasing emphasis on separation and independence. You and your child have a shared interest in seeing that diabetes is used as little as possible to negotiate these conflicts. Let your adolescent's rebellion be about not cleaning her room; at least that won't land the young rebel in the hospital. You can help keep your child's vital health interests from being a battlefield: be sensitive to changing emotional needs in adolescence, prepare to "give" on less crucial questions. For example, early adolescence is often a time of quiet introspection rather than highly structured activity. Children at this age may prefer listening to the stereo to participating in sports and music lessons. Realistically, you cannot expect a child with such inclinations to be gung-ho about exercise and blood sugar testing. However, you can and must expect the child to carry out the essentials.

When your child neglects his health, step in and set clear limits. Beyond this, give him a strong positive message about the value of good diabetes control and support him in maintaining as high a standard as is feasible in the context of other developmental needs. With all the denial adults with diabetes show, children can hardly be expected to be rational and realistic on their own, not when they are so susceptible to fantasy and to the influence of their social environment outside the home. Here as elsewhere, parental authority and guidance are called for. Make clear that, even if perfect blood sugar control remains out of reach, your child does have something to gain from maintaining good control. Then accept that the choice will ultimately be his own.

Parents Have to Live, Too

In the midst of caring for a diabetic child, parents must see that their own physical and emotional needs are not neglected. This is more easily said than done, especially in the harried weeks after onset. In Paul Kozlowski's words, "People have no idea what a strain this is on parents. It was four months before we could sleep late or go out for a drink together." In such an atmosphere tensions can accumulate. Although the Kozlowskis believed that the experience of caring for Amy had brought them closer together, they also noticed "a bickering, an edge in our voices, that wasn't there before." They found themselves snapping at each other: "Why don't you go get it?" "Yeah, okay, if you don't want to do it, I'll do it." It is good to be conscious of these tensions and to do something to reduce the pressure. You might see a counselor or (whenever feasible) enlist a trusted family member to help care for the child.

Mothers and fathers often react differently to their child's illness. Their knowledge and confidence may vary as well. Paul Kozlowski, already familiar with the disease (his father had had diabetes), remarked that "during the first couple of weeks I worried more about Mary than about Amy." He reacted more calmly than Mary did, even though he knew better than she how serious a disease diabetes is. Even as Mary learned more about it, she and Paul continued to disagree about many questions that came up. She insisted, for example, that any baby-sitter they hired be "a knowledgeable, competent person." He replied, "What does 'competent' mean – that they can dial a phone? Amy hasn't had trouble at night for a long time." Such differences of opinion, attitude, and temperament are normal and, as many couples will be quick to point out, not confined to diabetes. The Kozlowskis were able to resolve them without undue strain, as they became more confident about meeting Amy's needs, and as Mary learned what Paul already had some inkling of – namely, that "you can't control the world for the sake of diabetes."

Sometimes, though, conflicts between parents have more serious consequences. One parent may blame the other for the child's illness (because of heredity), or one parent may assume the role of "expert" while the other withdraws from participation and remains uninformed. One father took care of all of his six-year-old son's diabetic requirements. The boy's mother, meanwhile, kept a fearful distance. While the father was away on business the boy had an insulin reaction during the night. His mother gave him more insulin, and he ended up in the hospital. The physicians, predictably, berated the mother: "How could you do such a thing?" But their anger could not take the place of the professional counseling that this family needed.

One responsibility parents should share is insulin administration. To say, "You give him the shots; I'll manage his diet," is to risk having the child associate pain with just one parent. For this reason the Kozlowskis wisely took turns giving Amy her insulin.

What about the Rest of the Family's Diet?

Families differ in the extent to which they limit the availability of food. When sweets are kept out of the house (except to the extent needed to balance the insulin and prevent reactions), the child has less temptation to contend with at home and feels less deprived relative to other family members. The rest of the family gets to eat a more healthful diet, too. Still, household dietary restrictions generally make sense only when they are completely voluntary – that is, when everyone shares in the enthusiasm for good eating habits. Diabetes can raise the family's consciousness about nutrition, exercise, and good health generally. Out of this awareness can come a positive commitment to better health habits, including reduced sugar intake. But when an improved diet becomes a grudging sacrifice, probably more harm is done than good. Parents and children become martyrs, and the diabetic child pays a price in guilt. If anything, sibling rivalries touched off by this unnecessary deprivation can be worse than those that arise from the diabetic child's envy of what the others can eat. If the whole family moderates its taste for sweets, great. But all family members should be able to enjoy foods of their own choosing in their own home. As Mary Kozlowski put it, "Amy's the one with diabetes; we're not."

Perhaps most important, children whose home environments are tailored to their special dietary requirements are not learning to maintain those requirements for themselves in a larger, unregulated world. The Kozlowskis understood this point as well. In Paul's words, "When Amy walks out this door, the world isn't going to stop and accommodate itself to her diabetes." By teaching Amy to meet her own needs in a normal, diverse home environment, her parents provided a foundation for self-regulation in any environment. And that is the most valuable thing parents can do for a child who has diabetes.

For Further Reading

Johnson, R.W., Johnson, S., Kleinman, U., and Johnson, R. *Managing Your Child's Diabetes* (rev. ed.). New York: MasterMedia Ltd., 1995.

Lawlor, M.T., Laffel, L.M.B., Anderson, B.J., and Bertorelli, A. *Caring for Young Children Living with Diabetes: A Manual for Parents.* Boston, MA: Joslin Diabetes Center, 1996.

Loring, G. *Parenting a Diabetic Child: A Practical, Empathetic Guide to Help You and Your Child Live with Diabetes.* Los Angeles: Lowell House, 1993.

Siminerio, L. and Betschart, J.E. *Raising a Child with Diabetes.* Alexandria, VA: American Diabetes Association, 1995.

Wysocki, T. *The Ten Keys to Helping Your Child Grow Up with Diabetes: A Practical Guide for Parents & Caregivers.* Alexandria, VA: American Diabetes Association, 1997.

Sex, Sexuality, and Pregnancy

9

Having diabetes profoundly affects the most intimate experiences in life – those involved in sexual relations and bearing children. In addition, it can alter one's image of oneself as a sexual being and as an actual or prospective parent. It is in these areas that diabetes may be felt most keenly, undermining a person's sense of wholeness. Yet it need not do so. Sexual and parental fulfillment are increasingly within reach for a person with diabetes – given some care, imagination, and flexibility.

Sexual Issues in Diabetes

Diabetes affects a person's sex life and sexuality (that is, one's sexual image and self-image) in a number of ways. In the following sections we relate some typical experiences.

Embarrassment

One easily imagined (and generally avoidable) nightmare is having to reveal your diabetes the first night with your lover. Usually, by the time you initiate a sexual relationship, you will have spent enough time together for the revelation to have been made in other ways – going out to eat, for example – and the fear of its happening at an awkward moment is usually more of a problem than the actuality. However, it could conceivably work out otherwise. As one young man exclaimed, "Now I know what goes on with a junkie!"

Lack of Spontaneity

Diabetes structures one's life in a way that is incompatible with late-hour socializing and sexual spontaneity, especially for the single person. In this incompatibility lies the dilemma of adolescence and young adulthood – that of having to choose between responsible diabetes management and living a "normal" life. At the extreme, diabetes may appear to place such a damper on sex as to rule it out altogether. One woman reported hearing as a teenager that "diabetics don't do it." Education and counseling are essential to prevent or correct such misinformation.

Insulin Reaction during Intercourse

"What if I have a reaction while making love?" is a common concern – and, for some, a common occurrence. A thirty-year-old woman says, "I know there will be times when I'll have to say, 'Excuse me, I have to get up and get a Life Saver.' But it's embarrassing."

Clinicians differ on how easily prevented these inconvenient hypoglycemic episodes are, but many recommend having a snack first. A psychologist who is more concerned with precise blood sugar regulation believes that a person with insulin-dependent diabetes should always test his or her sugar before having sex. "It's no worse than putting in a diaphragm," he says. He describes a severe reaction he experienced once when he did not do so.

I was making love with my girlfriend in the middle of the night when I started to lose my erection. I began to question my desire for her until I realized what was happening. I excused myself, went to the bathroom, and got a blood sugar reading of 20. In other words, I shouldn't even have been conscious. But I was able to stagger to the kitchen for some orange juice. My

Sex, Sexuality, and Pregnancy

*girlfriend, who was familiar with my general diabetic require-
ments and procedures, didn't know what was happening until I
explained it afterward.*

A less systematic person might have skipped the test and gone
directly for the juice. The story does, however, point out the danger of mistaking an insulin reaction (often unrecognizable when it
first comes on) for a deficiency in yourself, your partner, or the
relationship. This is the opposite of another common problem discussed earlier – attributing all changes in moods or relationships to
fluctuating blood sugar levels.

Fatigue

Like any other exertion, sex is affected by the variations in energy
that a person with diabetes experiences. After some years with either
type 1 or type 2 diabetes, you may find yourself having sex less frequently as a result of intermittent fatigue. As a man in his early thirties explains, "I sometimes put it off because I feel crummy."

It is, however, important to distinguish between physical lethar-
gy, or other minor symptoms of diabetes, and the use of these
symptoms as an excuse to withhold sex from your partner. This is
an example of how diabetes can become a weapon of manipulation in family conflicts, as discussed in Chapter 7. Worse, it is not
always a simple matter to tell when this is happening because it
isn't necessarily conscious. When you don't feel at one with your
partner, you may "really" feel too tired for love-making, whether
or not you have diabetes at all. In any case, when you aren't up to
making love, an expression of affection can let your partner know
that it's the fault of your physical condition, not the relationship.

Oral Contraceptive Use

Oral contraceptives are generally a birth control option for women
with type 1 and type 2 diabetes. But oral contraceptives such as
steroid hormones can raise blood sugar through increased insulin
resistance. Regular blood sugar monitoring is essential. Oral

contraceptives are ruled out for women who have hypertension or some types of vascular disease.

Impotence or Decreased Sexual Function

A man's ability to have an erection may be temporarily impaired by either high or low blood sugar. Impotence is one of the long-term neurological complications of both kinds of diabetes and one of the most common complaints among diabetic men. Its incidence in diabetic men has been estimated at between 40 and 60 percent. Many of these cases, however, may be of emotional origin, just as they are in nondiabetic men. A study in which a group of diabetic men had their patterns of erection recorded while they were asleep found evidence suggesting that impotence was organically caused in 28 percent of the cases and psychologically caused in 28 percent (Fisher et al., 1982).

When related to diabetes, impotence is usually the result of impairment to both the nervous and vascular systems serving the male genital organs. Unlike many long-term complications, impotence does not seem to be related to how long a man has had diabetes. In its early stages, a man may first experience less rigidity and a decrease in frequency of erections. This can progress until he is not able to have erections at all. It is important to remember, however, that despite these problems, sexual drive is usually maintained.

Impotence has been one of the great "silent issues" in diabetes. Even when it is not a present reality, it (like blindness or amputation) can be an unspoken fear. It needs to be brought out in counseling relationships and support groups. Open discussion can help distinguish between cases of physiological and psychological origin so as to provide for proper treatment. It can also contribute to alleviating the intense despair a man may feel about sexual disability, which otherwise can undermine diabetes management and erode the will to live.

There is less of a problem for women with diabetes with regard to sexual functioning. The difficulty for younger women primarily takes the form of vaginal dryness during sexual activity.

Lubricants can help alleviate the problem. As a woman gets older, she may in addition encounter reduced sexual desire, more painful intercourse, and more difficulty achieving orgasm due to diabetes. A health care practitioner can discuss the possibility of estrogen as a therapy. Women, as well as men, should rule out the side effects of certain medications as contributors to sexual disability.

Both men and women who encounter decreased sexual function may benefit from consulting a specialist, alone or with their partners. The impact of sexual disability on marriages and other intimate relationships needs to be explored. Devastating as the experience of impotence can be, by no means does it close the door to sexual satisfaction. Both partners can reach orgasm even if the man does not have an erection (a man can ejaculate and have the sensations associated with ejaculation without being erect). Here a man in his mid-thirties who has had diabetes for twenty-five years describes how he and his wife compensate for his increasing sexual incapacity:

I've always had the feeling that I'm not as strong, not as well equipped physically as other men because of diabetes. But it wasn't till about halfway through my first marriage that I began to be unable to have erections on demand. This was stressful for me and my wife because I didn't know enough to attribute the problem to diabetes until after the marriage ended. Instead, "failure" became a self-fulfilling worry for me.

Over the years there have been more and more requisites for me to have sex. My diabetes has to be in perfect balance. I can't predict when I'm going to be able to have an erection. But I can keep it in perspective because intercourse isn't necessarily the best sex.

Women have told me that no one has made them feel the way I do. I can really get off on a woman's body and excite her orally, by touching – by making her feel loved. I've always enjoyed doing that. Now I can experience "failure" as physical, not personal, because my second wife gives me total acceptance as a human being who has diabetes.

If this kind of adaptation is not satisfactory, mechanical devices can be used to produce an erection. These create a vacuum and draw blood into the penis, at which point a band is applied to restrict blood outflow. In addition, a man can have his erectile capacity enhanced with vascular surgery to repair blood vessels, or he may consider a penile prosthetic implant. One type of prosthesis remains elongated, but can be bent downward like a straw; another is inflatable to simulate natural erections. Medications, which can be taken orally or injected directly into the penis, may be useful. Men will want to check with their doctors about whether the drug Viagra is appropriate for them. Treatment for impotence also includes improving blood sugar control and eliminating any medications that compound the problem.

Finally, it should be made clear that impotence, like other complications of diabetes, is by no means inevitable or universal. A woman who lived with a man in his fifties, who had had insulin-dependent diabetes long enough to suffer other complications, remarked, "He has the sex drive of an eighteen-year-old."

Excess Weight, Unattractiveness, and Avoidance

Part of the sense of loss that comes with the diagnosis of diabetes is the fear of losing one's sexual attractiveness. This loss may be seen as resulting from injection bruises, from disfigurement caused by anticipated complications, or from an intangible feeling of physical incompleteness or deficiency. Most typically, however, one feels unattractive because of being overweight. This is a problem in the sex lives of many people who do not have diabetes. It is also commonly associated with type 2 diabetes. Being overweight usually precedes and contributes to diabetes. And it may already have served as a way of avoiding sexual intimacy; in that case, diabetes simply becomes an additional excuse. A woman in her thirties, asked whether having type 2 diabetes interfered with her sex drive, replied:

No, I never had much anyway. I usually ate instead. Now, with the diabetes, I feel even more inhibited because I can't take

Sex, Sexuality, and Pregnancy

birth control pills. But it was never a big priority in my life. What you don't have you don't miss.

Losing weight brings an additional benefit: feeling – and being – more attractive to potential sexual partners. For some, though, the benefit is an equivocal one. That's why they don't lose weight. Sharon, forty-five years old, is overweight and has type 2 diabetes. Her case shows how the association between sexual problems, "unattractiveness," and diabetes can be just the tip of the iceberg. A deeper family conflict must be addressed if the diabetes is to be successfully treated.

Sharon had had several sessions with a diabetes counselor before she mentioned obliquely that she had "a problem with my husband that's connected with my health." She indicated that she felt some discomfort in talking about this "problem," and the counselor did not press her to do so. During a subsequent session, when the counselor asked about her marriage, Sharon revealed that her husband had "injured himself" fifteen years earlier and had since been incapable of sex. Lowering her voice, Sharon confided, "There's a lot of risk for me in losing weight. It's like a time bomb."

The counselor then explored with Sharon what seemed an obvious risk in her situation – namely, that if she lost weight she might begin to attract the attention of other men. She would then face choices that threatened to undermine her personal values and her marriage. Seen in that light, her excess weight may have been protecting her against unsettling and disruptive possibilities. Sharon, feeling vulnerable about this issue, again put off further discussion.

Later, however, she returned to the subject with a revelation that gave her problem a new dimension. "I'm not even so sure," she said hesitantly, "that the problem at home is my husband's as much as it is mine. I'm not so sure the situation couldn't be changed. If I lose weight, our sexual relationship might pick up again. And then I would have to start asking some questions." If her husband's impotence turned out to be reversible, then the long lapse in their sexual relations would no longer be safely attributable to an accident. The two of them would share responsibility for it – she for becoming unattractive to him, he for withdrawing from her. Sharon feared that this realization would lead her to feel angry toward her husband: "I'd have to ask him why he's been short-changing me all this time!"

Sharon's case may seem unusual, even unique, but it really isn't. Her story, with whatever individual variations, is that of any person with type 2 diabetes who needs to lose weight but does not do so. With so much to gain by losing weight, and so much to risk by not losing weight, what is the problem? What stands in the way? Each individual's situation is different; for example, a man may be afraid to compete with the memory of his athletic father. But somewhere at the root of the matter there is usually a story like Sharon's – a reason for being overweight even at the price of having diabetes.

It is important that Sharon's dilemma be articulated and consciously examined rather than allowed to sabotage the treatment of her diabetes. The prospect of reviving her sexuality, and with it the attentions of her husband and/or other men, has created an unconscious conflict which she can all too easily resolve as she has all along – by being overweight. Before she confronts her husband, Sharon needs to clarify her own values and preferences. What does she want from her husband sexually? What, if anything, does she want from other men? How much will she compromise to preserve her marriage?

Although the quality of her husband's participation in this exploration and in their relationship will be a factor in her choices, those choices and the responsibility for making them are still her own. Her self-esteem need not depend on her husband's acceptance or rejection of her. The better able she is to clarify her choices – and the fact that she has choices – the better able she will be to remove the unconscious impediments to weight loss. But to do this she needs support, and so she has turned to her diabetes counselor, just as others might turn to a physician, nurse, psychotherapist, friend, or diabetes support group. Whatever source of support one chooses, the acknowledgment and sharing of the dilemma are the first steps toward resolution.

Sex and the Insulin Pump

As the insulin pump and other continuous-wear devices for diabetes treatment are developed, the issue arises whether these implements interfere with sexual activity. This question will be discussed in Chapter 11.

Pregnancy and Childbearing

A woman who has diabetes today has virtually as good a chance to give birth to a healthy baby as any other woman. Pregnancy is one time, however, when tight blood sugar control (preferably with the aid of home blood glucose monitoring) is essential.

Despite the reassuring prospect of a normal outcome, pregnancy and childbirth raise large emotional issues when diabetes is already present in the family. These include long-range worries about heredity and childrearing as well as immediate concerns about the pregnancy itself.

Broader Issues for Prospective Parents

When a prospective parent has diabetes, he or she fears the hereditary risk involved in having children. Pregnancy can reactivate these fears. Without genetic counseling, the couple is likely to suffer the consequences of misinformation. Attitudes range from "What, me worry?" to the mistaken belief that diabetes is inherited in straightforward Mendelian fashion (i.e., that a child with one diabetic parent has a 50 percent probability of being diabetic). The actual figures (given in the previous chapter) are considerably more encouraging, but reality never stops parents from worrying. Parents who have diabetes, or who have had it in their family, typically watch a child's diet and test blood sugar even when the child has not developed diabetes. Earlier, they may have wondered whether they should have children at all.

If you are considering having a child, you may find genetic counseling useful, especially if you have a need for reassurance or feel there are special considerations or complications in your case. Weigh the decision carefully in light of your personal values. Keep in mind the data in Chapter 8. But keep in mind as well the ever-improving quality of life a person with diabetes can look forward to today. Keep in mind also the distinction between the facts (about the heritability of diabetes) and the subjective interpretation of the facts. One person's interpretation might be "If my child has diabetes, that would be just awful!" Another's might be "I've lived well with diabetes; my child could, too." Perhaps your interpretation would fall between these two extremes. No interpretation is right or wrong; any interpretation (unlike the facts) can be changed.

A person contemplating motherhood or fatherhood may also worry that diabetes will leave her or him with less energy for child-rearing and a shortened life span as a parent. A woman who might otherwise delay starting a family may feel pressured to bear children while she is young and in good health, before complications set in.

Concerns Surrounding Pregnancy

Despite the excellent odds of having a healthy baby, pregnancy and birth are not free of emotional concerns for a woman with diabetes. Blood sugar regulation, which must be maintained more vigilantly than at other times, is thrown off by the physiological changes of pregnancy. In effect, it must be learned anew.

Women with type 2 diabetes who take oral medications are sometimes advised to switch to insulin during pregnancy (itself a considerable emotional adjustment to add to the normal dislocations of pregnancy) to achieve tighter control and to avoid risks to the baby. When necessary, multiple daily injections are used to control hyperglycemia. Particular attention should be paid to hypoglycemia and ketosis.

Blood sugar control is essential, even in the first weeks after conception. Indeed, careful monitoring should begin as soon as pregnancy is planned, even before pregnancy is confirmed. Much of a baby's critical development – including heart, brain, spinal col-

Sex, Sexuality, and Pregnancy

umn, nerves, and muscles – occurs during the first six to eight weeks after conception. When diabetes is well controlled in early pregnancy, the chances of birth defects associated with diabetes drop dramatically. Near-normal glucose levels also lower the risk of miscarriage. A glycated hemoglobin test, which reflects average blood sugars over the previous weeks, can determine whether the time is optimal for getting pregnant. An unplanned pregnancy – in which blood sugar has not been well controlled – will certainly raise fears of possible birth defects.

The high cost of pregnancy for a woman with diabetes can be another cause of stress. Frequent tests throughout the pregnancy and extended hospitalization at the time of birth add up to a crushing financial burden, unless fully paid for by health insurance. In addition, depending on her condition during pregnancy, the doctor may advise reducing work hours, or stopping work altogether earlier than planned. This could put an additional strain on the family's finances.

Increasingly women are giving birth successfully under very difficult conditions. Still, pregnancy can aggravate a diabetic condition that may be developing and risks remain a serious consideration. A diabetic woman with vascular complications, for example, will be concerned about further damage to her system. "Will I survive?" "Will I go blind?" "Will the child be all right?" are especially intense questions at this time. A woman with cardiovascular disease may be advised not to become pregnant. A pregnant woman with diabetes may experience a temporary or permanent decrease in kidney function, and kidney disease is a significant risk factor. On the other hand, with treatment available today, her baby's chance for survival can be greater than 90 percent. A woman undergoing ambulatory kidney dialysis may be able to give birth under the careful attention of experienced specialists.

Diabetic retinopathy can develop rapidly or worsen during pregnancy. A woman with serious retinopathy may be able to have laser treatments before becoming pregnant or when the problem is detected. As a rule, however, a woman in an active phase of retinopathy may be advised not to continue a pregnancy, although she may be able to bear children subsequently during a quiescent phase. When one decides not to have children because of such a complication, it means mourning the loss of a basic fulfillment in life.

A Successful Pregnancy

Chapter 4 told the story of Denise, a young woman who had lived in a prison of secrecy throughout childhood and adolescence and well into adulthood. The decisive event that enabled her to free herself from this shame and deception was the birth of her daughter, Nancy.

Denise had been married a number of years when she and her husband decided to have a child. (Originally they resolved not to have children. At that time they, like the doctors who advised them, had overestimated the heritability of type 1 diabetes. They also did not have the benefit of recent medical developments that reduce the risk for both mother and baby.) Having turned thirty, and having reached twenty-five years of diabetes without complications, Denise found herself thinking about having a child. "If I could pull it off, I'd like to do it." One day, her husband turned to her and said, "You know, I've been thinking a lot about having a baby." "Me, too," she gulped.

Denise called her doctor, expecting him to say, "Oh, but what about your kidneys? What about this? What about that?" Instead, he said, "Fine, but do it right away." Thus began a process of detailed planning, all done with professional care and precision. Denise interviewed people she knew, read articles, sought referrals. A specialist told her, "If your eyes and your kidneys are normal, and if your blood sugar is in the normal range for the first three months, you have essentially the same chance of giving birth to a healthy baby as any other woman."

Denise could hardly believe it. "It didn't seem possible," she recalls. She and her internist discussed whether, during pregnancy, she should go on the insulin pump. He finally said, "I think you and I together can beat the pump" and recommended an obstetrician whose attitude was reassuring rather than alarmist. To Denise and her husband, the obstetrician's anticipation of "pretty much a routine pregnancy" was a welcome antidote to their own obsessiveness.

It seemed a miracle that Denise became pregnant almost immediately. "This baby wanted to be born," she said. She had what she calls "a textbook pregnancy: an active baby, insulin increased on schedule, all tests well in the normal range from beginning to end. Everything that happened confirmed that we had done the right thing at the right time." Denise had vaginal delivery after labor was induced at forty weeks. "Nancy was a big baby (nine pounds). She needed special care for a couple of days, but, in all respects, she was a normal child."

The experience of pregnancy was a positively reinforcing one for Denise. She and her husband had gambled and won. They would face life with diabetes with greater confidence, although (given her age) they would probably not take a chance on another child. Denise's doctor (who boasted to a leading medical authority about "beating the pump") was also affected by this positive spirit. "I don't see any sign of changes in your eyes," he told her, "and I don't think I will ten years from now." Most gratifying, as described in Chapter 4, was the effect on Denise's self-esteem and acceptance of her diabetes. Giving birth crystalized an important realization: she was strong enough to dispel the cloud of secrecy under which she had hidden this part of herself.

For Further Reading

Bartholemew, S. P. Make way for baby. *Diabetes Forecast,* December, 1997: 20–33.

Raffel, L. J. and Rotter, J. I. Genetic counseling for families of persons with diabetes mellitus. *Medical Aspects of Human Sexuality* 20(2) (1986):51–54.

Task Force for the American Diabetes Association Council on Pregnancy. *Diabetes and Pregnancy: What to Expect.* Alexandria, VA: American Diabetes Association, 1992.

Work and Play

10

Work, insurance, medical costs, travel and recreation, drug and alcohol use – these, like food and exercise and family life, are the stuff of everyday life. Coming to terms with the impact diabetes has on each of these areas makes a great deal of difference to the quality of life one can enjoy. We will discuss only the most important issues involved, because (unlike the emotional and personal issues raised in previous chapters) these matters are well covered in other books listed at the end of this chapter and at the end of the book. Organizations such as the American Diabetes Association, as well as organizations specifically concerned with disability issues (also listed), offer printed and online guidance on these practical questions.

Job Performance and Job Discrimination

Type 2 diabetes usually does not (except in some cases when treatment with insulin is required) seriously hinder a person's working life. It most often appears at a time in life when one is well established in a career, and it does not noticeably detract from one's performance – indeed, it may not be noticeable at all until complications arise. Type 2 diabetes usually has no apparent symptoms and is not characterized by metabolic instability. Dietary restrictions might set one apart when eating at work, but the same could be true for any person who is dieting.

With type 1 diabetes, the need to take insulin – and the possibility of insulin reactions and diabetic comas – can make diabetes a visible presence in the workplace. (Because hypoglycemia is a more acutely severe and unpredictable condition than hyperglycemia, some people deliberately keep their blood sugar running on the high side to avoid detection at work – a very unwise strategy in the long run.) The need for precise coordination of diet and insulin makes flexible scheduling of work difficult. The journalist covering a story whenever it breaks, the counselor in a crisis atmosphere, the truck driver making long hauls through the night, the factory worker on the night shift tempted by breakfast twice a day – all must make special adjustments so that their job does not interfere with their diabetes management or vice versa. Some people find it difficult to work in an environment where they cannot stop to have a snack when they need it.

Employers may be concerned about inflexible scheduling, the effects of physiological fluctuations on energy and work performance, and sick days. However, none of these considerations justifies a policy of job discrimination against people with diabetes. Rather, they should be dealt with on an individual basis. There is no reason, for example, to assume that a person with diabetes will take more sick days than anyone else. Physicians who keep their diabetes well controlled have been more than equal to the demanding schedule and high responsibilities of their profession. Ken Dugger excelled at the strenuous life of a federal law-enforcement agent, ready at a moment's notice to travel with his diabetes supplies (Mazur, 1995). One can do just as well in any calling. Recent research confirms the reports of experienced observers, going back over decades, that people with diabetes rate better than average in work performance and reliability (Greene and Geroy, 1993).

The American Diabetes Association takes this position concerning employment: "Any person with diabetes, whether insulin dependent or non-insulin dependent, should be eligible for any employment for which he/she is otherwise qualified." The struggle against prejudicial discrimination has been a long one, however, and it is still going on. The Rehabilitation Act of 1973 protected people with disabilities, including those associated with diabetes, from employment discrimination on the part of the federal government or companies receiving federal funding. In 1990 the Americans With Disabilities Act (ADA) extended this protection to civilian employees of companies that employ 15 or more people. Persons who come under the protection of these laws are not required to reveal to their employers that they have diabetes, except as necessary to benefit from the provisions of the law.

The Americans With Disabilities Act

The Americans With Disabilities Act provides that employers must make reasonable accommodations for the disabilities of employees who are qualified to perform the essential functions of the job. Reasonable accommodations for a person with diabetes might include exemption from shift rotations; work breaks to test blood sugar, eat a snack, or go to the bathroom; and permission to keep food and diabetes supplies near the work area. If there is no infirmary or other specialized area that can be set aside for insulin injection, a person's privacy should be respected when using the rest room for this purpose. Employers need not, however, accommodate insulin injection in a public work area. Questions of space such as these can be negotiated individually or through collective bargaining.

The extent to which absences and lateness should be accommodated depends on whether they occur for medically necessary reasons and whether the essential requirements of the job are defined so as to include reliable attendance and promptness. Employers have the right to hold disabled individuals to the same performance and behavioral standards as any other employees. Indeed, the great majority of people with diabetes want nothing more than to show that they can meet those standards. Sometimes, however, it is difficult to determine what is misbehavior and what is a direct consequence of a disability. In one case, a U.S. Court of Appeals ruled that an employee fired for absences associated with diabetes was fired solely because of his disability, rather than for misbehavior, under the provisions of the ADA (*Teahan v. Metro-North,* 1996). To get his job back, however, he would still have to prove in court that his frequent absences could be reasonably accommodated by his employer. Where frequent absences become an issue on the job, a person with diabetes may seek assistance not only under the ADA, but also under the Family and Medical Leave Act (FMLA) of 1993, which allows workers up to 12 weeks of unpaid leave each year to attend to their own or family members' serious illnesses. An employee who exhausts this leave allotment under FMLA may be entitled to additional leave under the ADA, provided that the employee remains qualified to do the job.

As anyone who has experienced the emotional consequences of chronic illness can attest, a serious chronic illness often brings with it some degree of psychiatric disability (Bursztajn, 1993). It can be a challenge both for employers and for the courts to distinguish between disruptive behavior that merits termination and visible signs of a mental impairment covered by the ADA. Further complicating the choices for someone who feels discriminated against on these grounds are the stresses of going through the legal process, which can aggravate whatever emotional problems already exist (Bursztajn, 1985).

In 1997 the Equal Employment Opportunity Commission (EEOC) issued guidelines for reasonable accommodations to be made for psychiatric disabilities under the ADA. Implementation is another matter. It takes nearly a year, on the average, for the EEOC to process a complaint, and the EEOC receives hundreds of complaints for every lawsuit it files. In some cases, however, filing a complaint with the EEOC may be a requirement for bringing legal action on one's own.

If you lose your job for reasons related to your diabetes, you may want to apply for disability benefits to make up for the lost income. Beware, though, of this "Catch-22": by applying for benefits, you may lose your right to sue as a victim of discrimination under the ADA. Some courts have accepted the contention of employers that a person who applies for social-security or private disability benefits is thereby admitting that he or she is not qualified for employment and therefore is ineligible for protection under the ADA. Fortunately, depending in part on the timing of the application for benefits, the courts appear to be moving toward a compromise position which allows people who have applied for permanent disability benefits to show that they are still qualified to do a particular job.

The courts will rule a disabled employee *not* qualified, however, if he or she poses a "direct threat" to the health or safety of others in the workplace, or to his or her own health or safety. (Even then, the employer must determine whether a reasonable accommodation can remove the threat.) For example, a court ruled that a chemical process operator with diabetes posed a direct threat to the work environment because of the possible consequences of a loss of concentration resulting from acute complications of diabetes (*Turco v. Hoechst*, 1996). Such determinations can be reasonable if they are made on a case-by-case basis. However, as diabetes activists are quick to point out, the blanket federal employment bans that still exist are inconsistent with the intentions of the ADA.

Not long ago, anyone found to have diabetes was immediately discharged from the armed services. Even now a person with diabetes cannot enlist, but someone who is diagnosed after enlisting may be able to stay in the military, depending on the type of diabetes, the medications required, and the person's service duties. A person with type 1 diabetes, if retained, will not be deployed worldwide. In civilian life, Ken Dugger fought successfully (both in court and by showing he could hold similar jobs in other federal agencies) to overturn the automatic exclusion of people with type 1 diabetes as U.S. Treasury agents (Mazur, 1995). In 1996 the Federal Aviation Administration rescinded its ban on recreational pilots' licenses for people with type 1 diabetes and began issuing licenses on a case-by-case basis. Heartened by this precedent, activists have campaigned against the federal regulation disqualifying people with type 1 diabetes from driving commercial vehicles in interstate commerce. In states that do allow them to drive commercial vehicles within state borders, people with type 1 diabetes have compiled an above-average safety record (Mawby, 1997).

Discrimination in Schools

Section 504 of the Rehabilitation Act of 1973 prohibits discrimination against people with disabilities in federally funded programs, including the public schools. Children with diabetes are also covered by the Individuals with Disability Education Act (IDEA) of 1990, which guarantees "free appropriate public education, including special education and related service programming for all children with disabilities." Parents who are concerned about their child's diabetes management in school, or about whether their child is getting the full school experience, can work with the school to develop a Section 504 plan or an Individualized Education Plan (IEP) under IDEA. (The school can apply for federal aid to help pay the extra costs of an IEP.) The plan may include provisions analogous to workplace accommodations, such as access to food and the bathroom, assistance with blood glucose testing or insulin injection, allowance for absences, and full participation in school activities. If the school authorities are not responsive to reasonable parental efforts to meet a child's needs, and if all efforts at explanation and negotiation fail, the parents may choose to take administrative or legal action.

Opposing Discrimination

Despite legal protections, discrimination (overt or subtle) still occurs. Stories like the following, told by a teacher in his thirties, are common:

> When I applied for one job I was told that I would have the job if I took a physical exam. I got through the exam without telling the doctor I had diabetes. Then I confided in the doctor, and I was not hired. Another time, when two of us were passed over for promotion, the other guy pursued it through channels as a case of discrimination on grounds of diabetes, and he ended up with a better job.

Sometimes diabetes is used as a pretext to reinforce discrimination on other grounds. A woman who joined the state police was disqualified from being a state trooper because she had diabetes, even though there were male diabetic troopers on the force.

Some manuals advise job-seekers to acknowledge their diabetes to employers and prospective employers, to build a record of credibility and good performance for the benefit of others who have diabetes. This is a case where what is best from the standpoint of public morality may not be best for the individual concerned. A woman who has worked in a number of public agencies warns, "Don't advertise your limitations to your employer." Similarly, the broad dissemination of accurate information about diabetes is a worthy effort, one that would seem all to the good. But a person whose employer is not fully aware of the degenerative complications of diabetes may well think twice about volunteering this information.

If you or someone in your family faces diabetes-related discrimination at work or in school, the *American Diabetes Association Complete Guide to Diabetes* (1996a) provides useful guidelines, resources, and steps to take. These are summed up by the motto: "First educate, then negotiate, and last, litigate" (p. 375).

Necessary Adaptations

Serious long-term complications may, of course, necessitate major adjustments in one's working life. According to the American Diabetes Association's guidelines on employability, the effects of complications (e.g., impaired vision, loss of limbs) on eligibility for employment should be evaluated without regard to the presence of diabetes. These effects include both the impact of the physical impairment on work performance and the loss of time for repeated surgical procedures (as in diabetic retinopathy). The same individualized evaluation should apply to an acute complication such as hypoglycemia, which has been used as a basis for job discrimination (ADA, 1998a).

Whatever the disability, one can always work. It may, however, take time to find suitable work, as well as to mourn the loss of one's previous career. Before facing up to that loss (whether temporary or permanent), one may go through a great deal of denial. A woman who worked in a government office suffered severe retinopathy with almost total vision loss, first in one eye and then in the other. (Her vision was later restored.) Concealing her condition from her employers, she did not miss a day of work, although she was reprimanded for being "moody"! A former nurse took a job as a medical assistant after she had become legally blind. After a week of deception and awkwardness she resigned for the good of the patients whose records she could only pretend to read.

Complications of diabetes may require adaptation in work as in other areas of life. People with vision loss have made successful transitions from paperwork to work emphasizing personal contact. A salesman with an amputated limb might become an office manager (if such jobs are available). One type of work available to people with a wide range of employment backgrounds is helping others – for example, as a diabetes counselor. People go into the helping professions for a variety of motives – to be of service to others, to learn about oneself and perhaps alleviate personal problems, and to exert some control over an uncertain world (Edelwich and Brodsky, 1980). Any or all of these motives may be powerful ones for a person who has experienced diabetes and its complications. A psychologist who leads diabetes groups and conducts research on the behavioral aspects of diabetes tells how his personal and professional lives have run together:

When I developed diabetes in my mid-twenties I had not worked in the area before, but my academic background had obvious relevance. "Aha!" I thought, "I can do something with this." I volunteered as a research subject and learned as much as I could. Working in the field has been therapeutic for me, in that it has given me a professional rationale for closely monitoring my metabolic state. Moreover, I can hardly teach adolescents to maintain good blood sugar control if I don't do it myself. I'm concerned about my credibility in their eyes as well as my own.

Work and Play

Insurance and Disability Payments

"Diabetes," a prominent physician once stated, "is the death knell insurancewise all over" (Rubin, 1982). Indeed, until the mid-1940s, insurance companies automatically rejected all applicants who had diabetes. Since then the situation has improved as insurers have become more discriminating about the impact of diabetes (in different forms and at different stages) on insurance claims from one type of policy or another.

Life insurance is becoming available to people with diabetes as life expectancy improves. However, affordable individual health insurance can be difficult to find for a person with diabetes. Fortunately, group insurance policies are usually open to all employees at a standard rate, regardless of health status. The Americans With Disabilities Act requires that an employer that provides health insurance must make the same policies available to all employees. People with diabetes who leave their jobs have been assisted in maintaining continuity of health insurance coverage by the Consolidated Omnibus Budget Reconciliation Act (COBRA) of 1985 and the Health Insurance Portability ("Kennedy-Kassebaum") Act of 1996. Special group health insurance and group term life insurance for people with diabetes have been available through organizations such as the Diabetes Group Insurance Trust. Medicare and Medicaid are additional options for those eligible. Overall, about 92 percent of adults with diabetes have some form of health insurance, leaving some 640,000 people without coverage (National Diabetes Data Group, 1995, p. 591).

Once you have health insurance (or if you are fortunate enough to be able to choose between plans), find out which of the many expenses involved in diabetes a plan reimburses. In the patchwork of policies and jurisdictions that now exists (with different minimum coverages mandated in different states), plans vary greatly in their coverage of supplies such as syringes and blood glucose monitors, as well as new treatment technologies such as the insulin pump and penile prosthesis. Many elderly persons who could be more self-sufficient with prefilled syringes have had only temporary coverage for these, and home care has been available to them only when acutely needed. On the other hand, having diabetes may entitle a person to reimbursement for procedures that others must pay for, such as treatment of ingrown toenails. A major point of contention has been reimbursement for education in self-management, which the American Diabetes Association (1998d) calls an essential component of good clinical care.

Managed Care

By far the most significant development in health insurance in recent years has been the emergence of managed care. When Health Maintenance Organizations (HMOs) introduced prepaid, fixed-premium health insurance coverage in the 1970s, this model had great appeal for people with an expensive chronic illness such as diabetes. By standardizing clinical procedures, HMOs often do better than private practitioners at preventive monitoring, accessing information in patients' records, and incorporating the findings of clinical research into daily practice. For example, HMO staff may be more likely to look up when you had your last eye exam, and thus discover a complication before it becomes more difficult to treat. Nonetheless, as HMOs have evolved into one form of managed care, a darker side of the picture is coming into focus. By limiting benefits, putting medical decisions in the hands of claim reviewers, and giving physicians incentives not to order certain tests and treatments, managed care has in some cases undermined trust between doctor and patient, compromised the decision-making process, and denied coverage for treatments recommended by the physician and chosen by the patient. Patients subjected to this heavy-handed cost cutting have ended up feeling alienated, hopeless, or angry (Bursztajn and Brodsky, 1996).

As noted in Chapter 6, research to date has not given any clear indication that the quality of diabetes care in managed-care settings is either better or worse than in traditional fee-for-service practices (Peters et al., 1996). Looking to the future, can managed care respond to the challenge posed by the Diabetes Control and Complications Trial (DCCT)? Judging from the experience of the DCCT, the intensive management required to achieve cost savings in later years from reduced complications of type 1 diabetes could cost an additional $4000 annually per patient (Quickel, 1994). Given the ultimate cost of complications such as heart disease, hypertension, and retinopathy, that investment is well worth making (Gilmer et al., 1997). Similar estimates of cost-effectiveness have been made for type 2 diabetes (Bloomgarden, 1996b). Managed-care organizations can realize substantial financial benefits from intensive treatment by looking to their long-term rather than short-term self-interest.

Managed care is evolving rapidly, and in unknown directions. Attempts to curb its excesses and protect patients' and physicians' prerogatives through legislative and legal action make it even more difficult to predict what managed care will look and act like even a few years from now. Meanwhile, if you believe that your treatment choices are being unnecessarily restricted by managed care, see if your doctor, nurse, or social worker will engage in a dialogue with you and act as your advocate within the plan. If you cannot get satisfactory results, consider changing plans (if possible) or finding out whether any state or federal laws or regulations exist to protect your right to make treatment choices.

Other Forms of Coverage

Accident insurance is another battleground in the struggle to remove discriminatory barriers. Buoyed by a Danish study showing that people with diabetes are no more accident-prone than the general population, diabetes advocates are opposing the practice of restricting coverage or charging higher premiums for people with diabetes (Mathiesen and Borch-Johnsen, 1997). Related difficulties have been reported with disability payments and educational assistance.

Individuals with severe visual impairments have been denied Social Security disability insurance payments because they are not legally blind. Unable to earn a living in ways they are accustomed to, not yet retrained for other work, they live in limbo, dependent on welfare until their vision deteriorates sufficiently to make them eligible for payments. A young woman who developed retinopathy without severe vision loss had a four-year college education subsidized by her state's bureau of vocational rehabilitation, to help her provide for herself if she should subsequently develop vision loss. Later, by then legally blind, she applied for assistance in obtaining a doctorate for the sake of job security, but was denied this help because she already had a master's degree – a kind of limbo of eligibility. If you find yourself in this situation, you may be able to get assistance from organizations for the blind listed under "Useful Resources" in the back of this book or from your state's commission for the blind. Knowing these pitfalls exist, you can plan ahead, make your needs known, and assert whatever rights you do have.

Diabetes Activism

When you walk into the waiting room of a diabetes treatment center, you are likely to find on the table (along with informational pamphlets) a flyer saying "Diabetes-Related Bill – TAKE ACTION! Write to your state legislator." Open a copy of *Diabetes Forecast,* and you'll see an appeal to "Sign this petition to the President of the United States! Increase funding for diabetes research." This grass-roots mobilization, on the successful models of AIDS and breast cancer activism, is a response to the problems people with diabetes face with discrimination and insurance reimbursement, and it is getting results at both the federal and state levels. Delegates for Diabetes, an advocacy training program started in 1995 by the American Diabetes Association (ADA), attracted 8000 volunteers in its first two years. To add your voice, contact the ADA or your local affiliate and ask for the staff person responsible for advocacy.

The Cost of Diabetes

Medical costs are a major – but often unacknowledged – practical and emotional issue for people with diabetes and their families. The following estimates have been reported to us as examples of the range of medical expenses associated with diabetes. They are approximations subject to change. Although medical expenses tend to rise with and even beyond inflation, the costs of new technologies may decrease as the latter become more commonplace and more easily produced.

For Amy, the four-year-old girl in Chapter 8: $60–70 a month for supplies (including $18 for syringes), plus two $30 physician's visits a month and special dietary foods. Medical expenses are covered by insurance, but for Amy's parents "the check isn't there when we need it."

For a woman who underwent periodic hospitalizations during a six-month period, including eye surgery and a kidney transplant (the latter $37,000 in itself): $150,000, covered by Medicare and Blue Cross/Blue Shield supplemental insurance.

For the total costs of pregnancy and childbirth for a woman with diabetes: $ 12,000–20,000, with about $800–1,000 paid out of pocket.

For Anne, the adolescent in Chapter 6 who left her family doctor (at $15 a visit) to go to a modern diabetes treatment center: $250 for a complete initial examination at the center ($100 of which was the doctor's fee), covered by health insurance with a co-payment.

For test strips for home blood glucose monitoring, 45 to 60 cents apiece, plus $250–400 for a meter if desired.

For an insulin pump, $1,000 to $2,800 plus the cost of home blood glucose monitoring.

Although people with type 2 diabetes usually do not have to bear the costs of insulin administration, they still incur the expenses of doctors' visits and of equipment and supplies for blood sugar monitoring (on top of the costs of other chronic medical conditions often associated with type 2 diabetes). The costs of supplies can be especially burdensome for the elderly on fixed incomes, who cannot choose to do without syringes and needles when prices rise steeply (as they sometimes have in recent years). The monetary cost of having diabetes in the family can be an unspoken cause of marital and parent-child conflicts. Parents under severe economic pressures have to be careful that these do not lead to resentment of a diabetic child.

Fortunately, there are ways to cut the cost of diabetes. Start by checking out the American Diabetes Association's annual *Buyer's Guide to Diabetes Products*. Test strips used for blood glucose monitoring can be purchased in bulk and can be cut into halves or thirds – a substantial saving if you test several times a day. Shop around for syringes; prices vary. Pharmacies make a great deal of money from diabetes; see if you can find one that will agree to a discount "bulk rate" for a regular customer. Finally, although this is not now standard policy, check with your doctor about the possibility of safely reusing disposable syringes.

In the managed-care era there has been a growing interest in estimating the costs of diabetes for society as well as for the individual and family. According to a 1992 study, annual health-care expenditures for a person with diabetes averaged more than three times as much ($9,493) as for a person who did not have diabetes ($2,604). In that year people with diabetes constituted less than 5 percent of the U.S. population, but accounted for nearly 15 percent of total health-care expenditures (Rubin et al., 1994). If the costs of lost productivity resulting from complications were added to direct medical expenses, the total might run close to $100 billion (National Diabetes Data Group, 1995, p. 601).

Recreation and Travel

Many stories throughout this book, particularly those told in Chapter 5 about the dilemmas of type 1 and type 2 diabetes, portray choices that must be made in the realms of friendship, active sports, and travel. Will a child with diabetes feel comfortable participating fully in sports in school and in the neighborhood? Can a childhood friendship withstand the strange rituals and restrictions of diabetes? How can an adolescent negotiate the conflicting demands of responsible diabetes management and "being one of the gang"?

For the parents of a child with diabetes, social life may seem to lose much of its spontaneity. "It hits me in the evening, when I'm feeling active," mused one conscientious mother. "I can't remember what it was like not to have to worry about having meals on time when we went out at night." Her husband added, "We can't go to the beach for a whole day or go out in the evening on the spur of the moment. We can't be delayed in traffic without thinking about Danny's needs. Maybe it would be that way with any kid, maybe not."

Those with type 2 diabetes need to get involved in some sort of regular exercise (it may be competitive sports). This often means breaking lifelong habits of inertia. One needs to shape one's social life so that it no longer revolves around food. This is difficult in a society that reinforces unhealthy habits of eating and drinking.

A woman whose husband has type 1 diabetes comments,

We can't take a vacation trip with a bunch of other people, because our needs are different from theirs. And to vacation alone together for a week or more is a real test of our ardor. You never go on vacation from diabetes; you always take it with you. For me a vacation used to mean sleeping late, eating too much or too little and at odd times. All that's out the window; we punch a time clock when we're away just as we do at home.

On long-distance trips punching the clock is more complex. Meals and insulin schedules must be coordinated with changes in time zones. Travelers also worry about needing medical care in a strange place, being stopped at an airport and questioned about injection apparatus in one's luggage, and running out of syringes and needles on a prolonged trip (this was not a problem a generation ago when one would carry a sterilizer rather than disposables). In some places it may be a challenge to find suitable food or potable water. One woman recalls her frustration on a trip to Europe at a time when "there was no sugar-free anything there."

Despite these difficulties, diabetes is becoming less and less of an obstacle to active recreational pursuits – including skiing, mountain climbing, and the like – and wide-ranging travel in the jet age. New resources are available – for example, a quarterly newsletter called *Diabetic Traveler.* Specialty Group Cruises offers cruises tailored for people with diabetes, with workshops on traveling safely with diabetes provided on board by the Joslin Diabetes Center.

Of course, there are many pleasurable activities that do not pose any special problems for people with diabetes, such as movies (without the popcorn), plays, museums, dancing, and country walks. Beyond these, the added motivation to keep fit, especially with type 2 diabetes, can open up new areas of enjoyment and personal growth. Toward that end, the International Diabetic Athletes Association was founded in 1985 to educate people with diabetes on the benefits of regular exercise and how to exercise safely (Thurm and Harper, 1992). How one can live a full life with diabetes is the subject of several excellent books listed at the end of this chapter and at the end of the book.

Alcohol and Drug Use

In a society in which eating luxuriously is the norm, it is sometimes said that people who have diabetes must be more virtuous than anyone else. The same is true with alcohol and drugs, which are an established part of our social environment, even while their abuse has visibly destructive consequences. For those who do not want to give up alcohol altogether, it can be included in a diabetic diet as a fat exchange. Care must be taken, however, to monitor and compensate for the effects of alcohol in combination with food as well as with insulin or oral medications. Alcohol can have a destabilizing effect on blood sugar, precipitating either hypoglycemia or hyperglycemia depending on the conditions under which it is used. Heavy drinking can exacerbate kidney failure and cause liver damage, which in turn may increase the severity of insulin reactions. A person who passes out from drinking may have an undiagnosed, untreated insulin reaction while unconscious. Indeed, people who take insulin wear identification bracelets because there is often diagnostic confusion between drunkenness and severe hypoglycemia.

Clearly, alcohol has the potential to complicate diabetes in several ways. Nevertheless, a study of people who had survived over fifty years with insulin-dependent diabetes revealed a variety of patterns of alcohol consumption, ranging from abstinence to moderate regular use (Cochran et al., 1979). Since numerous studies in recent years have shown that moderate alcohol consumption helps prevent heart disease, those moderate regular users may well be benefiting from their drinking. Individuals at risk for ischemic heart disease show the greatest reduction in mortality resulting from drinking, and people with diabetes are at high risk for ischemic heart disease. Therefore, people with diabetes (especially type 2) should not be discouraged from drinking moderately (Bell, 1996).

Since diabetes provides young people with legitimate access to injection supplies and experience in their use, might not some use these supplies to "mainline" other drugs, especially in view of the emotional stresses an adolescent with diabetes experiences? (Such stresses also contribute to alcohol abuse.) While having diabetes does facilitate drug abuse for some young people, others who abuse drugs by other means avoid mainlining because of its unpleasant associations ("I take enough injections already"). It is probably most accurate to say that some people who use illicit drugs happen also to have diabetes and that drug abuse in conjunction with diabetes can have especially serious consequences.

Len developed diabetes at the age of ten. He quickly learned to take his own insulin shots so that he could go about his life freely. His parents, feeling guilty and unsure about how to handle him, spared him from discipline on grounds that he required special attention. Len manipulated this attitude, using diabetes as "the excuse no one would argue with, at home or in school. Whenever I didn't want to do something, whenever I wanted to put something over on people, I could always cop to the diabetes."

Diabetes did not create this manipulativeness in Len; he reacted to diabetes as his early experiences had taught him to react to life in general. The urge he felt to "get something out of" people is commonly observed in narcotic addicts, and indeed Len began using heroin in his late teens. With it he covered up his feelings about having diabetes. "I could push the heroin button and 'not have diabetes' for the next several hours," he says. Meanwhile, he carried his manipulative approach into his work. A gifted business promoter, he would "work incredibly hard, swing some big deals, get people appreciating me, and then disappear for a while and do my own thing."

Len went on this way for ten years until his drug habit grew to such proportions that he was unable to work. His judgment impaired, he suffered a serious overdose. He then realized that he had to quit if he wanted to go on living. On top of everything else, heroin is "cut" (diluted) with sugar, which increased his need for insulin to a degree that was difficult to measure. Now drug-free, Len must not only restabilize his metabolism, but also revive his business career, in the hope that it will give him a satisfying outlet for his manipulative energies and independence.

In retrospect, Len sees an interesting and poignant connection between his two self-injection routines. Having diabetes taught him that he needed the needle, needed a chemical in his body to give him life. For him, injecting a drug was not an unnatural thing to do, but the reverse. To inject a different drug for a different purpose was not a big step. It was "like just pushing a different button."

Illicit "recreational" drugs like marijuana and cocaine also complicate diabetes management. Among other effects, marijuana provokes a craving for sweets, and cocaine triggers the release of sugar stored in the liver into the bloodstream. Although it would be better if people did not use these drugs, some rational, productive, otherwise law-abiding people do use them, and some of these people have diabetes. Leaving aside questions of morality, the issues for people with diabetes who are considering drugs are: first, what harm does anyone stand to suffer from these drugs; second, what special harm does a person with diabetes suffer? Having acknowledged the facts and the probabilities, one must make a choice. If the choice is to take drugs, the task is to negotiate this (just as with normal alcohol use) so that it will have the least possible destructive consequences. If you are thus inclined,

Work and Play

look for a doctor who is willing to enter into this kind of exchange:

Patient: I have occasionally used cocaine.
Doctor: I recommend against it under any circumstances.
Patient: If I should take it again, what are the main dangers, and how can I compensate?
Doctor: It releases sugar into the blood. Try to compensate by taking more insulin and not eating at the usual time. Test your blood sugar frequently and carefully. Let me know what you come up with, and we'll work something out. Just remember, it would be better if you didn't use drugs at all.

Here the doctor does not abandon the patient just because the patient is doing something the doctor does not approve of. This kind of trusting relationship, applied here to a sensitive area, honors the patient's personal values, the doctor's ethical responsibilities, and the stake both have in the patient's health. For the "patient" in this scenario – a "person" once outside the doctor's office – this is one more creative adaptation to a complex illness in a complex world.

For Further Reading

American Diabetes Association. *American Diabetes Association Complete Guide to Diabetes: The Ultimate Home Diabetes Reference.* Alexandria, VA: American Diabetes Association, 1996a: 375–398.

American Diabetes Association. *Buyer's Guide to Diabetes Products.* Alexandria, VA: American Diabetes Association [published annually].

Baker, B. Taking it to the states: insurance reform sweeps nation as grassroots movements spur state legislators to action. *Diabetes Forecast* May 1997: 44–48.

Dawson, L.Y. *Managing Diabetes on a Budget*. Alexandria, VA: American Diabetes Association, 1995.

Gillespie, S. How to win with your insurance company. *Diabetes Forecast* December 1994:42–47.

Gordon, N.F. *Diabetes: Your Complete Exercise Guide*. Champaign, IL: Human Kinetics Publishers, 1993.

Graham, C., Biermann, J., and Toohey, B. *The Diabetes Sports and Exercise Book: How to Play Your Way to Better Health*. Los Angeles: Lowell House, 1995.

Hornsby, W. (Ed.). *The Fitness Book for People with Diabetes: A Project of the American Diabetes Association Council on Exercise*. Alexandria, VA: American Diabetes Association, 1995.

Mazur, M.L. Fighting back. *Diabetes Forecast* August 1995:16–22.

Mohr, M. Have you heard about COBRA? *Diabetes Forecast* December 1994:63.

Stoneham, L. Health insurance: more options, more opportunities: educating companies to cover test strips, preventive care. *Real Living with Diabetes* March–April 1995:6–8.

Thurm, U. and Harper, P.N. I'm running on insulin: summary of the history of the International Diabetic Athletes Association. *Diabetes Care* 15 (suppl. 4) (1992):1811–1813.

Technology and Its Limits

11

Before the discovery of insulin in 1921, life with diabetes was short and grim. Even with a near-starvation diet, one could not hope to survive for very many years. But those who stayed alive long enough to see the beginning of insulin treatment saw a new world of hope open up, one in which they could have something approaching a normal life and a normal life span. We may be on the verge of similar breakthroughs today. New methods of diagnosing, treating, or preventing diabetes and its complications are being discovered that may again transform the experience of having diabetes. The prospect of benefiting from these advances as they become available gives added incentive to take good care of yourself in the meantime. Still, it is important to keep a realistic perspective on what *any* technology can do, to avoid disappointment and disillusionment.

What the New Technologies Are

Much has been learned regarding diabetes in the last decade. Monitoring has improved enormously, and with tight glucose control there is great hope for delaying or even eliminating the complications of diabetes, living a healthier and longer life, and living a more "normal" lifestyle. Researchers are seeking ways to achieve increasingly precise blood sugar regulation without the need for multiple daily injections. The externally worn insulin pump delivers a constant flow of insulin that can be adjusted to mimic natural variations in the secretion of insulin by the pancreas (for example, by increasing the dose at mealtimes). The pump in current use is called "open-loop," because it cannot by itself measure the need for insulin and adjust the dose accordingly. This must be done by the person wearing it, with the help of home blood glucose monitoring.

"Closed-loop" pumps, which detect fluctuations in blood sugar and adjust the insulin dose automatically, currently take the form of consoles used for hospitalized patients. A great hope for the future, and a challenge for current research, is a closed-loop pump with miniature glucose sensors. Since the pump is in constant contact with the bloodstream, this could provide instantaneous or continuous blood sugar monitoring without the pain and inconvenience of finger pricking. Implantable closed-loop pumps show preliminary promise but are not yet available.

An alternative strategy is to restore natural secretion of insulin through transplantation. Pancreas transplants have been performed successfully but have a high rejection rate, and the side effects of antirejection drugs predispose the recipient to severe infection and possible cancers. Presently, pancreas transplants are recommended only for those in need of concurrent renal transplants, for whom the risk of immunosuppression is considered more acceptable.

Sometimes an entire pancreas is taken from a cadaver; sometimes a portion of a pancreas from a living donor closely related to the patient is used instead, because it is less likely to be rejected. The patient's own pancreas is left in place. As a rule, it can still produce digestive enzymes, and this function can continue uninterrupted whether or not the transplant is accepted.

Instead of transplanting all or part of a pancreas, some researchers are attempting to transplant insulin-producing beta cells, or islets (clusters) of these cells, into veins going into the liver. The cells can be treated to prevent rejection. Islet cells have been successfully transplanted from one species of animal to another, thus raising the hope that animal cells can be transplanted to human beings. At this time, islet cell transplantation is an experimental procedure.

While we await these replacements for the daily dose of insulin, research continues to see which route for insulin delivery most closely approximates the physiological effects of normal secretion by the pancreas. Several routes allow for sufficiently rapid absorption to control the rise in blood sugar at meal times. The most promising, because of its convenience, is the nose. Nasal insulin nebulizers (spray devices) require further development, however, to become a reliable delivery mechanism. In the meantime, new devices called insulin "pens," with premixed insulin stored in prepared cartridges, make it easier to take several injections a day.

Recent developments in insulin include new formulations as well as the use of insulin in combination with oral medications to enhance its effect and lower the insulin dose. Human insulin (Humulin) is produced by recombinant DNA technology. Its advantage over its predecessors (beef and pork) is that it does not produce allergic reactions because the immune system is not sensitized to it. Another encouraging development is the recent release of lispro, a rapid-acting insulin used with the pump. Annie is a 42-year-old woman who, after using the pump for six years, switched to the fast-acting insulin and discovered a new psychological freedom. "The effects of the long-acting insulin were more volatile and unpredictable. Now, with the fast-acting insulin, I can eat and exercise with hardly any worry." Since the bolus of insulin is dissipated in an hour, she is at little risk of hypoglycemic reaction when she exercises. The immediate effect, followed by a fast flushing out, of the insulin has freed her from fear of insulin shock and given her greater control over her life. "Instead of all the effort and confusing details associated with injections, I can push a button in a restaurant and snack freely."

A variety of other technological advances are beginning to make it possible to improve blood sugar control, prevent (possibly) or cope with complications, and make life with diabetes less difficult and more "normal." The management of diabetes has been revolutionized in recent years by the self-monitoring of blood glucose. Home blood glucose testing has replaced urine glucose testing for most people with type 1 and type 2 diabetes. (Urine ketone testing remains an important part of monitoring, particularly in people with type 1 diabetes and pregnant women with type 1, type 2, and gestational diabetes.) Community-based intervention programs have been effective in substantially increasing the number of people with diabetes who self-monitor (American Diabetes Association, 1996c). But one of the major disincentives to self-monitoring, the pain associated with repeated finger pricking, is still unresolved. Stanley (who in Chapter 5 discussed how he came to terms with the need to lose weight) describes the problem without hiding his frustration:

> I know that frequent blood glucose testing – up to several times a day – is recommended for tight control, but the fingers can get quite sore from all that pricking. You hear people say, "I don't test. My fingers are already raw." Then they have poorer control and a poorer prognosis. Scientists lose touch with people in the trenches – the nurses and especially the patients and families. We want researchers to give more thought to everyday usage and make technologies more user-friendly. People who don't have diabetes are looking for Nobel Prizes by trying to identify the genes for diabetes. Why not devote more research funds to practical discoveries? With a reasonably priced, relatively painless test, people would have better control and live longer with fewer complications.

In answer to this evident need, noninvasive, convenient testing that would facilitate more frequent monitoring is on the horizon. One device being tried out pricks the skin on other parts of the body, thereby avoiding the fingers. Such technologies as radiation, fluid extraction, and closed-loop pump monitoring systems could potentially monitor blood glucose levels on a continuing basis. Tactile techniques for home blood glucose monitoring that enable visually impaired people to regulate their own blood sugar are already available.

Home blood glucose monitoring is a proven tool for better control, but only if one makes use of the test results. Otherwise, daily testing may be a waste of money. One study suggests that for people with type 2 diabetes, 4–5 tests a week are adequate (Bloomgarden, 1996a). Another suggests that for patients with type 2 diabetes not treated with insulin, home blood-glucose monitoring "is no more effective but 8–12 times more expensive than urine testing in facilitating improved glycemic control" (Allen et al., 1990).

The glycated hemoglobin test provides aggregate blood sugar readings over the previous few months, as opposed to moment-by-moment "snapshots." This broader measure of metabolic well-being is very useful in type 2 as well as type 1 diabetes and leads to fewer long-term complications. The test, performed in a doctor's office or clinic, should be repeated every 2–6 months. By measuring the concentration of hemoglobin molecules (which are found in red blood cells) that have glucose attached to them, the glycated hemoglobin test complements day-to-day-testing. It is a relatively simple but powerful way to assess blood sugar control.

Other technologies offer new hope as well. For example, laser surgery enables some individuals who have diabetic retinopathy to regain lost vision. For men who are impotent, penile prosthetic implants are among the devices that allow for a restoration of sexual functioning (see Chapter 9).

When we think of new technology for treatment of diabetes, we should not think only of those developments that are obviously biomedical, or "technological" in a narrow sense. New discoveries about food may prove at least as important as the invention of new gadgets. Current recommendations on nutrition have become more flexible. Now, in place of a strict set of guidelines, the emphasis is on individualized treatment focusing on metabolic outcomes. Dietary exchange lists are being revised with the discovery that carbohydrates with similar amounts of calories and nutrients are absorbed into the blood at different rates of speed and therefore have different effects on blood sugar. The same foods may influence blood sugar differently depending on the combinations in which they are eaten. A high-fiber diet is taking on greater importance and may turn out to be a major factor in the treatment of type 2 diabetes.

Oral medications, too, are changing. Research is focusing on combining the oral medications with one another and with insulin to best control blood sugar. The "second generation" of oral hypoglycemics (sulfonylureas) can now be used in smaller doses with less risk of side effects and fewer potentially harmful interactions with other drugs. The four categories of oral medications currently available are the sulfonylureas, which promote insulin secretion by the pancreas and may improve insulin sensitivity; the biguanides (metformin), which decrease the liver's production of glucose, improve insulin sensitivity, and improve lipid cholesterol profile; troglitazone, which primarily improves insulin sensitivity in muscle and fat (it requires some insulin to be present to function); and acarbose, which delays carbohydrate absorption. Capoten (or captopril) is among the group of medications known as angiotension converting enzyme inhibitors (ACE inhibitors). ACE inhibitors treat high blood pressure, protect the kidneys by decreasing protein loss and maintaining kidney function, improve insulin sensitivity, and improve lipid cholesterol profile.

Behavioral "technologies," when they can be shown to make a difference, represent an appealing alternative to medical technology (Cox and Gonder-Frederick, 1992; D'Eramo-Melkus et al., 1992; Glasgow et al., 1996; Smith et al., 1997). Stress-management techniques, such as those presented by Herbert Benson (Benson and Proctor, 1994), are being studied for their impact on blood sugar control. Such behavioral methods may make insulin or oral medications unnecessary for some people with type 2 diabetes, although this effect is not yet well documented.

Research in genetics and immunology also has a contribution to make to diabetes treatment – and perhaps prevention (Polonsky et al., 1996; Raffel et al., 1996; Turner and Levy, 1996). As the gradual (or "smoldering") development of diabetes is observed in close relatives of diabetic individuals, we begin to learn how genetic vulnerability manifests itself in autoimmune reactions that destroy insulin-producing cells. As this research progresses, immunotherapy may become a reality in the treatment of diabetes, including anticipatory treatment in genetically high-risk individuals monitored from an early age for the appearance of destructive antibodies.

Finally, computer technology can assist greatly both in patient education and in the collection, storage, and retrieval of clinical data. With all the measurement and recording routinely involved in diabetes care, the computer's capacity to retain, organize, and display information selectively is a great boon to the human beings who must ultimately interpret the information. Computers can be used in the patient's home, the doctor's office, or both together. It is exciting to think that a patient can enter a daily dietary log and test results into a personal data file and send it electronically to the doctor's office, where the patient and doctor together can review it at the patient's next visit.

Hope is an important ingredient of good care and emotional health. At the same time, hope must be tempered with caution. Newspaper accounts emphasize the most hopeful future possibilities, not the side effects of new treatments or the years of animal and human studies that lie ahead before a new device or technique can be made available to the public. Physicians working on the technological frontier may, in their enthusiasm and their desire to attract volunteer subjects, unwittingly encourage unrealistic expectations. An educator and advocate asks, "Do we need a study on the diabetic's tolerance for dashed hopes?"

New solutions, however valuable, bring new problems, and maybe some old ones, too. No one would feel anything but thankful for the life-saving discovery of insulin, for example, but probably no one at the time anticipated the complications that would appear fifteen years down the line, now that people with diabetes live long enough to experience them. Here was a great blessing – and with it a new set of problems requiring a new set of solutions. These solutions in turn are to be sought with enthusiasm and hope, but with a realism that anticipates further problems as well.

Expectations versus Limitations: The Case of the Insulin Pump

Improved blood sugar control will prevent, retard , or even reverse complications of diabetes, and the insulin pump has been demonstrated to afford improved metabolic control for many users. But these benefits will remain speculative until the pump has been in use longer. The pump can have medical side effects ranging from skin irritations and infections at the needle site to machine malfunctions, and some physicians contend that it has not proven itself any more efficient than multiple (four) daily injections of insulin. On the other hand, with a supply of insulin available at one's fingertips and with use of the fast-acting insulin, the pump can allow for greater flexibility in scheduling meals, work, and exercise.

Annie, who earlier described her enthusiasm for the fast-acting insulin, says that all but one of the people she knows who use the pump are "deliriously happy. The benefits of the insulin pump over intensive four-shots-a-day treatment don't get documented in comparative research. The movement toward the pump is not so visible, but the profits of the company that makes the pump are rising. Physicians are not being educated about the experience of using the pump. They see only quantitative studies. They don't see the convenience and they certainly don't see the potential. There could be a glucose sensor connected to the pump. Think of the possibilities!"

Currently the pump appears to be used mainly by achievement-oriented individuals seeking to better their already excellent control and, at the other extreme, by those who have not attained a satisfactory degree of control without it. There is a large group in the middle – those whose blood sugar is in reasonably good control – who are not availing themselves of the benefits the pump might offer. One must be highly motivated to use the pump, for it requires considerably greater attention and effort than the standard injection routine. In return for this hard work it yields measurable results, which some people find very satisfying. Doing more can be less of a burden when you are doing it yourself, with a sense of freedom, responsibility, and accomplishment.

Like other medical technologies, the pump was developed and bestowed on a grateful world without regard for the psychological adaptations it would entail, which have had to be worked out in practice. For example, a person who has not accepted having diabetes may be pushed to an emotional crisis by the necessity of acknowledging it constantly (by wearing the pump) instead of just

Technology and Its Limits

taking two injections a day and forgetting about diabetes the rest of the time. A major emotional issue with the pump is its visibility, which signifies public acknowledgment and the risk of stigmatization. Concerns about attractiveness and sexual image may be one reason why fewer women than men appear to be using the pump. One man decided, "It's for me, so I don't care what anybody sees." A woman joked, I have to fend off the punks in the subway who eye my pump, thinking it's a Walkman." These attitudes are changing now that Nicole Johnson has been crowned Miss America while wearing an insulin pump. Her efforts are bringing about greater public understanding and acceptance of the pump.

Even so, an overly upbeat presentation of the pump, one that shows only the bright side, risks loss of credibility with those who look below the surface. One man who was interested in using the pump declined the opportunity to participate in an experimental program because the physician who sought to recruit him denied that any patients were having psychological problems. "He wasn't being straight with me," this man said. Given the positive results (physiological and psychological) that the introduction of the pump has, on balance, thus far achieved, those who favor the pump need hardly fear presenting the full picture.

Joe is a thirty-year-old married man who has had type 1 diabetes for twenty-two years. He has been on the insulin pump for one year, and his experience with it reveals complexities that overenthusiastic advertising glosses over. Joe, who was selected for the pump because he was seen as a stable, responsible person, was not given psychological counseling in preparation for the new treatment. He was told that it was not a cure-all and that he would have to work at achieving control, but he was not prepared for the sheer amount of work he would have to do or for the discomfort the needle in his stomach would cause him. "It blew my mind for a few weeks," he said. "At times I wondered whether the whole thing was worth it." By "the whole thing" he meant not just the pump, but living with diabetes at all. Ironically, the clinic at which he obtained the pump had psychological services available, yet even in his worst moments of despair Joe neither sought nor was offered counseling. He might have benefited from being more assertive. Yet along with his despair he felt uncomfortable at the idea of talking with anyone about such intimate concerns.

In retrospect, Joe believes that his expectations about the pump were "about three-quarters accurate." He expected that he would feel better, which he does "only to a degree. At least the highs and lows are more moderate." He expected that blood sugar control would be easier than before, when actually it requires more effort than two shots a day. He expected that there would be no pain, but in fact the needle hurts when he bends over, sleeps on it, or is "hugged the wrong way." At first he had numerous bruises caused by the tape allowing the needle to move, but he has obtained a preparation that reduces the inflammation.

Joe is concerned about visibly identifying himself as diabetic by wearing the pump. However, since he works in a human services occupation, people who see the pump often assume it is a beeper. (Most people are too preoccupied with their own affairs to be curious about the pump.)

Sexually, Joe has found the pump inhibiting. "If I were nineteen or twenty and dating," he reflects, "the sight of a needle in my stomach might be a problem for women – it might seem gross." As it is, his wife can handle the sight of it, but it takes a lot of humor and teasing for the two of them to negotiate the awkwardness of working around the pump when they make love.

A couple can schedule sex every two days when the needle is taken out and replaced, but then they would lose spontaneity. If the needle is in place, the couple must experiment with positions. With the stomach as the site, it may be easiest for the man (if he is the one wearing the pump) to lie on his back, the position that involves the least movement on his part. If the needle goes into the leg, as it does in another variation of the pump, there may still be problems with sex, although not in precisely the same way.

When asked whether he raised sexual questions at the clinic when he was given the pump, Joe exclaims, "God, no! Who would talk to a doctor about that?" This reticence is all too common on the part of both patients and physicians. But despite these and other problems, Joe is pleased to have the pump and is committed to staying with it. Soon he will be switching to the fast-acting insulin that has worked so well for Annie. "Let's see how that works," Joe says.

Imagine what we would think if insulin injections had been invented after the pump. "A medical breakthrough!" the newspapers would trumpet. "New freedom and mobility for diabetes sufferers! People who have been carrying around a box with a needle in their skin twenty-four hours a day can now control their blood sugar with two daily injections." This kind of fantasy keeps technology in perspective. Should careful use of the pump turn out to prevent, delay, or lessen the chance of complications, the extra work it entails may well be worth it. Meanwhile, pump versus injections is one more choice to be made on the basis of probabilities and personal values (see Chapter 5).

There is good reason to greet the insulin pump enthusiastically and, for many, to consider using it. But there is also reason to share Denise's satisfaction (in Chapter 9) at having "beaten the pump" during her pregnancy, or to note that in one test a patient given thirty-five hours of intensive education and $2.50 worth of blood testing strips achieved closer control with less insulin than a $60,000 artificial pancreas (Rasch, 1982). There is a place for skepticism as well as for hope. We can pause in celebrating the march of science to understand the woman, already carrying a glass eye and a transplanted kidney, who, when asked how she felt about the pump, replied, "Thanks, but no thanks. I've got enough spare parts!"

For Further Reading

American Diabetes Association. *American Diabetes Association Complete Guide to Diabetes: The Ultimate Home Diabetes Reference*. Alexandria, VA: American Diabetes Association, 1996a (paperback, 1997).

Benson, H. and Proctor, W. *Beyond the Relaxation Response: How to Harness the Healing Power of Your Personal Beliefs*. New York: Berkley Publishing Group, 1994.

Nathan, D.M. with Lauerman, J.F. *Diabetes: The Most Comprehensive, Up-to-Date Information Available to Help You Understand Your Condition, Make the Right Treatment Choices, and Cope Effectively (A Massachusetts General Hospital Book)*. New York: Times Books, 1997.

Saudek, C.D., Rubin, R.R., and Shump, C.S. *The Johns Hopkins Guide to Diabetes: For Today and Tomorrow (Johns Hopkins Health Book)*. Baltimore: Johns Hopkins University Press, 1997.

Support Groups

12

Physicians and other medical professionals often lack the time, skill, or inclination to deal with emotional issues. Friends and family have their own preoccupations, their own emotional investments in situations. So where can one turn for emotional support and guidance? More and more, the gap is being filled by support groups. These groups for people with diabetes and their families may be billed as "therapy" or "self-help," and they may be established at the initiative of treatment professionals or patients. Either way, they provide a forum for self-expression and an opportunity for practical and emotional education.

Besides adding a dimension of support that is often missing from medical treatment, groups help overcome the isolation that keeps people who have diabetes from sharing common experiences and learning from one another. The guardedness, even secrecy, with which many individuals treat their diabetes is a barrier to getting to know others who have the disease. Some people actively avoid such contacts. They don't want to be reminded of diabetes, or they don't want to be typed as "invalid" or "handicapped." As one observer noted,

For many patients it appears that seeing – or even hearing of – another diabetic has the effect of looking into a mirror, and not liking it. Yet, this is not without conflict; there is real ambivalence in the feeling, "Well, I'm not alone," and "He can really

understand me," coexisting with anxiety about a common fate. (Frankel, 1975)

Support groups are designed to bring out the positive side of the ambivalence, the nourishing feeling that "Someone else has felt the same way I have – and survived."

This chapter will provide some guidelines about what to look for in a group and what to expect (as well as what not to expect) from it. If there are no groups in your area that meet your needs, use these guidelines to start your own!

Types of Groups Available

A typical group is open to anyone who has diabetes, type 1 or type 2, including any complications that do not prevent a person from getting to the group sessions and participating fully, and any emotional problems that do not disrupt the group (as it might, say, if someone regularly showed up under the influence of drugs). Such groups allow participants to learn from others with any type or stage of diabetes and to see universal human concerns beneath varied circumstances. Other groups serve the specialized needs of individuals with type 1 or type 2 diabetes, children or adolescents, insulin pump users, those who have particular complications such as diabetic retinopathy, parents of diabetic children, and so forth. People who have diabetes can also benefit from groups with a focus other than diabetes and its complications, such as weight reduction (in type 2) or living with chronic illness.

For those whose participation in groups is hindered by geographical remoteness, an inconvenient work schedule, or physical disability, online discussion groups such as the one maintained by the Joslin Diabetes Center offer an alternative. Access to the Internet removes barriers of space and time, making some form of contact (if not the full experiential processing of a well-led group) available at the user's convenience. A person who feels uncomfortable with face-to-face interactions about diabetes may choose initially to join an online group, which may then serve as an entry point for more direct participation later.

Online chat groups can be located on the websites of major organizations such as the American Diabetes Association (listed at the back of this book), or on the major Internet-access services. These sources also provide paths to diabetes newsletters, some of them existing only in electronic form, which reflect various lay and professional viewpoints. A woman who credits these resources with greatly facilitating her adjustment to diabetes says, "A lot of the advice on the Internet is better than what you get from physicians, but don't believe everything you read."

Unrealistic Expectations, Real Benefits

Don't come into a group thinking that it will solve your problems. A group cannot do what nature, the health care system, your family and social support network, and your own emotional resilience and recuperative powers are unable to do. It can, however, help you mobilize all these resources. Participating in a group will not make you a "good diabetic" (as if that goal had any meaning). If you come into the group depressed, don't expect the group, by itself, to get you out of the depression.

What, then, can you really expect from a group? First, a group serves as a catalyst for identifying practical needs and getting outside help (e.g., from public service agencies) where necessary. (This is a major purpose of groups dealing specifically with severe disabilities, such as vision loss from diabetic retinopathy.) Second, it provides an opportunity to express feelings and air personal experiences in an atmosphere of empathy and nurturance. Third, it offers emotional support in coming to terms with illness and disability. Many constructive and innovative adaptations can grow out of identification with others who have similar problems. From this identification come new perspectives, new hope, and new energy to live with – but not for – diabetes.

Note that this process of imitation and influence is mutual. You teach even while you learn. On the one hand, you gain hope and encouragement from other members of the group. On the other, you experience yourself as strong and purposeful as you give the same support and comfort that you receive. In a well-run group, the participants inspire one another to be more active and energetic and achieve the fullest possible involvement in life.

Can being in a group lead to improved blood sugar control and a better medical prognosis? Yes, although that is not the primary purpose of a support group. For example, at the psychosocial unit of the Joslin Diabetes Center in Boston, involvement in groups over a period of time has for some individuals been associated with improved metabolic functioning. Why does this happen? As we noted in Chapter 3, emotional balance can affect diabetes control in two major ways. First, feelings of well-being and connectedness with others are linked with reduced stress, which in turn may have directly beneficial physiological effects. Second (and less speculatively), a positive emotional outlook enables and empowers one to care for oneself responsibly. Not surprisingly, then, groups designed to build coping skills have been shown to be effective in improving diabetes control as well as emotional adjustment (Jacobson, 1996b; Rubin and Peyrot, 1992). Research has confirmed the value of group support in coping both with day-to-day problems in living with diabetes (Anderson et al., 1989) and with serious crises and complications (Bernbaum et al., 1989).

Groups foster responsible self-care by focusing attention on the major barrier of *denial* and allowing members to work through it in a nonpunitive atmosphere. One member of a group may avoid blood sugar testing so as not to see the evidence that she really has diabetes. Another may "forget" to take insulin at inconvenient times. Another may take excessive does of insulin, as if that would suppress the diabetes altogether. A fourth may munch on cookies during the group sessions. By coming together in a group, these individuals, all in different corners of the same boat, can support one another in confronting and overcoming their denial. In the Joslin groups, for example, some individuals decided they wanted improved control badly enough to justify the added effort of going on the insulin pump.

Issues Worked Out in Groups

In addition to the question of denial, support groups deal with the range of emotional and practical issues discussed throughout this book. Groups commonly begin with a venting of anger against physicians – a useful starting point, but not a place to get stuck. Family issues – conflicts with parents, sibling rivalries, dependency versus autonomy – are replayed in groups, with other group members and the group leader unwittingly placed in the roles of absent family members. Once dramatized in the group, these issues can be examined consciously, long-held attitudes and perspectives challenged, and emotional energies redirected. Group members learn how they and their families have used diabetes as a pretext for avoiding issues and maintaining habitual patterns of interaction.

Sibling rivalries in groups often break down into "good patient-bad patient" conflicts and competition for the group leader's (parent's) attention. In one group a woman brought in blood-testing equipment and wanted to test everybody to show that she had the "best" blood sugar. The group as a whole may adopt this false elitism as a defensive posture: "We're good, healthy diabetics. We take care of ourselves. We don't want anybody with complications." This attitude is part of the material to be explored by the group for self-awareness. It should not dictate a policy of "drawing the wagons together" and closing off the group to new people, problems, and emotions.

The following examples illustrate the range of situations that come up in groups:

Case 1: A prison guard who was facing surgery for complications of diabetes was pursued by an inmate with a knife. He stopped the attacker by feigning an insulin reaction. In this situation, as brought out in group discussion, the guard had played out both his fear of surgery (the knife) and a tendency to use diabetes to ward off threats.

Case 2: A woman with type 2 diabetes had to take insulin during an illness. Despite the inconvenience and discomfort, she was inwardly pleased by this development because it made her feel more completely a part of a group in which everyone else was taking insulin. Group discussion focused on her need for belonging and the desirability of strengthening other human connections in her life.

Case 3: The mother of an adolescent child feared that she would no longer be an adequate parent as her vision deteriorated from diabetic retinopathy. The group mourned this loss with her and worked with her to distinguish between what she could do for herself or her child and what she would need to have others do. The group also relived with her the miracle of motherhood and the joy of having a healthy child. While helping her adapt to the reality she faced, the others in the group shared her past and present dreams.

Guidelines for Support Groups

Groups are not for everyone. A person's capacity to benefit from a group depends on an ability to communicate verbally and to establish supportive relationships in the group. It depends as well on an intention to use the group to cope and help others cope with diabetes (as opposed to having love affairs, forming an exclusive club, complaining, or scapegoating doctors and nurses). If you are in doubt about whether you or someone else can benefit from a group at a given time, this question can be explored in one-to-one counseling.

The emotionally turbulent period immediately following diagnosis may not be the best time to get into a group; individual sessions with a counselor may be more appropriate for a while. Likewise, it is not necessary to stay in a group forever. You may need to meet added demands on your time made by work, school, or family; you may feel that you have reached a stable emotional resolution; or you may not want to go over the same issues with new people after a period of heavy turnover in the group. The purpose of the group is served when you can take what you have learned and apply it in "real life" (Edelwich and Brodsky, 1992).

Groups typically meet for one and one-half to two hours weekly or biweekly. New members may be asked to commit themselves to stay for at least eight to ten sessions. After that the group can be open-ended, with each individual deciding when to terminate. Serious commitment can be encouraged with a contract by which one pays for one's place in the group at each session whether or not one attends.

In a group billed as therapeutic, trained leadership is essential. It is not important whether the group leader is a psychiatrist, social worker, physician, nurse, technician, or lay person. It is important, however, that the leader be trained in the principles and methods of group therapy, including focusing and interpreting discussion and providing information when appropriate (Tattersall et al., 1985; Yalom, 1995). Such trained leadership is the main difference between therapy groups and self-help groups organized by and for lay persons, which work by mutual support and example alone.

Occupying a broad middle ground between group psychotherapy and mutual self-help is a practical approach to group counseling outlined elsewhere by the authors (Edelwich and Brodsky, 1992). While designed for groups led by trained counselors, this model can be adapted for self-help groups if participants take responsibility for creating a group experience that is more than socializing or "ventilating" feelings. Neither psychodynamic nor educational in a didactic sense (as lectures and films are), this "group process" has a task-oriented focus in an atmosphere of emotional immediacy. The group is a microcosm of real life, with the facilitator setting the group climate, dealing with the resistance that naturally and inevitably occurs, and modeling genuineness, trustworthiness, responsibility, respect and concern for others, empathic responses, and appropriate confrontation and self-disclosure. Group members develop problem-solving and decision-making skills as they identify and clarify issues in their lives that require intervention. In so doing, they become better able to manage their lives outside of the group.

A group that is to be more than a private club, especially one sanctioned by a treatment facility, has a responsibility to accept new members who meet basic criteria for eligibility consistent with the stated purpose of the group (provided that there are places open). Those who resist new members may need to be reminded of the underlying principles of sharing and mutual support from which they themselves have benefited. It is reasonable to ask someone to leave the group – not because of personal dislike or rivalry (which is material to work through) – but for disruptive behavior or failure to keep agreements with the group.

Groups vary as to how broad a membership they encompass. Those with a narrowly restricted membership have certain tactical advantages. For example, children and adolescents may feel more free to talk about drugs, sex, and parental conflicts in a group limited to their peers. Women can use an all-female group to share concerns about sex roles, marriage, and childbearing. However, in the absence of vigilant leadership, groups with an obvious badge of membership tend to encourage an "'us' against 'them'" mentality, whether "them" signifies doctors, people of a different age or gender, or people who don't have a particular complication. Being with people of different ages, genders, and medical histories exposes participants to various points of view and shows that issues such as isolation, abandonment, and fears about the future are universal human dilemmas. Radical as this sounds, it may be advantageous to invite a doctor or nurse into the group, not as a one-time guest, but as a regular participant. The presence of a professional on equal terms with lay persons can turn a grievance session into a constructive exchange. The broader the membership, the better the group can prepare each member to survive – and thrive – in a larger world.

For Further Reading

Edelwich, J. and Brodsky, A. *Group Counseling for the Resistant Client: A Practical Guide to Group Process.* New York: Lexington Books, 1992.

Tattersall, R. B., McCulloch, D. K., and Aveline, M. Group therapy in the treatment of diabetes. *Diabetes Care* 8 (1985): 180–188.

Yalom, I. D. *The Theory and Practice of Group Psychotherapy* (4th ed.). New York: Basic Books, 1995.

The following organizations are among those that offer support services. Addresses can be found starting on page 296. See also the web sites starting on page 291.

American Diabetes Association
Federation for Children with Special Needs
Joslin Diabetes Center
Juvenile Diabetes Foundation International
National Association for the Visually Handicapped (NAVH)
National Federation of the Blind
Vision Foundation, Inc.

Glossary

Acetest – A type of test strip material used to indicate sugar level in urine.

Acetones – Fatty acids produced during improper metabolism of body fat.

Acidosis – A condition in which excessive amounts of ketone acids are present in the blood.

Adrenal – A gland which manufactures and releases essential hormones, including adrenaline.

Adrenaline – A hormone secreted by the adrenal glands (or produced synthetically) which stimulates the nervous system.

Alpha Cells – Type of cells in the pancreas responsible for producing the hormone glucagon.

Amniocentesis – A test of the fluid surrounding the fetus which helps to determine whether certain diseases or conditions are present.

Antibiotic – Any of several drugs that have the ability to destroy bacteria in the body.

Artery – A blood vessel which transports blood away from the heart.

ATPase – An enzyme, found in all body cells, which allows normal energy production.

Beta Cells – Type of cells in the pancreas responsible for the production of insulin.

Blood Glucose Level – The amount of sugar (glucose) present in the blood at a given time. Normal blood glucose levels range between 70 and 140 milligrams per centiliter of blood.

Carbohydrates – The sugars and starches found in food (such as breads, fruits, and potatoes) which are easily utilized for fuel by the body.

Cardiovascular System – The body's circulatory system, which includes the heart and blood vessels.

Cataract – A condition of the eye in which the lens becomes cloudy.

Clinitest – A type of test strip used in testing urine in order to approximate blood sugar level.

Coma – Condition of deep unconsciousness.

Cornea – Clear, central part of the eye through which light enters.

Diabetologist – A doctor who specializes in the treatment of diabetes.

Diabinese – Type of oral medication consisting of chlorpropamide, effective in lowering blood sugar level.

Diuretic – Type of medication which causes the loss of excess fluids; with the use of a diuretic, more urine is secreted.

Enzyme – A protein produced in all cells which speeds up chemical reactions in the body.

Fat – A type of fuel for the body derived from foods such as meats, dairy products, and vegetable oils.

Gangrene – Death of body tissue resulting from poor blood supply in a particular area.

Gene – Unit responsible for inheritance found in all living organisms.

Gestational Diabetes – Any degree of glucose intolerance that begins or is first noted during pregnancy.

Glucagon – A hormone, produced by the alpha cells in the pancreas, which raises blood sugar through the process of breaking down glycogen.

Glucose – A form of sugar, usually blood sugar.

Glucose Tolerance Test – Test used to determine the presence of diabetes. Demonstrates the blood sugar response to a quantity of glucose given by mouth.

Glycogen – The bodily storage form for carbohydrates (glucose) found in the liver and muscles.

Glycosuria – The presence of glucose in the urine.

Hormone – A chemical substance produced in the glandular cells of the body (or manufactured synthetically) which stimulates other body cells.

Hyperglycemia – A condition in which the blood sugar level is higher than normal limits.

Hyperinsulinemia – A condition in which an excessive amount of insulin is present in the blood.

Hypersmolar coma – A condition in which a very high blood sugar level is associated with severe dehydration and altered mental status.

Hypoglycemia – A condition in which the blood sugar level is lower than normal limits.

Hypoglycemic Agents (Drugs) – Medicines taken by mouth which help to reduce the blood sugar level.

Hypoglycemic Reaction – Condition resulting from drop in blood sugar level to amounts far below normal. Symptoms can include hunger, nausea, weakness, and confusion.

Impaired Fasting Glucose and *Impaired Glucose Tolerance* – Conditions in which the blood sugar level is above normal, but not high enough to meet diagnostic criteria for diabetes.

Insulin – A hormone produced in the pancreas and secreted into the blood, where it regulates the body's sugar absorption.

Insulin Pump – Machine which injects insulin automatically and regularly into the body.

Insulin Reaction – Common complication experienced by persons with diabetes in which the blood sugar level is lower than usual due to overtreatment of insulin or oral hypoglycemic medicines, inadequate food intake, or exceptional exercise.

Insulin Resistance – Condition in which an immense insensitivity to insulin occurs.

Islands of Langerhans – Clusters of cells located in the pancreas which include the beta cells, where insulin is produced.

Keto-acidosis (ketosis) – Condition in which ketones are present in the blood and urine due to high blood sugar level.

Ketones – Fragments of fatty acids which are the end products of improper fat breakdown. Ketones occur as a result of the incomplete burning of body fat for energy.

Ketonuria – Condition in which ketones are present in the urine.

Kidneys – Organs in the body responsible for filtering blood and chemical wastes.

Laser Treatment – Therapy for retinopathy using light rays which may help to reduce bleeding and thus improve sight.

Medic Alert – Type of identification (card or bracelet) indicating the presence of a disease (such as diabetes) and emergency precautions.

Metabolism – Process, including all physical and chemical changes occurring in the body, in which food is broken down and used to provide energy necessary for maintenance and growth.

Nephropathy – Renal (kidney) disease.

Neuropathy – Any disease of or associated with the nerves.

Ophthalmologist – Doctor who specializes in treatment of the eye and of diseases related to the eye.

Oral Hypoglycemic Medicines – Substances taken by mouth which help to reduce blood sugar levels.

Pancreas – Gland located near the stomach which secretes insulin into the blood.

Phenformin – A type of oral hypoglycemic medication, used to lower blood sugar levels.

Podiatrist – Doctor who specializes in the treatment of the feet and of disorders related to the feet.

Prediabetic – Occurring before the onset of diabetes.

Retina – Membrane area at the back of the eyeball (inside the eye) which receives light and images.

Retinopathy – Disease of the eye specifically concerning the retina.

Self-Monitoring – Active and frequent testing (of blood and urine, for example) to control diabetes.

Stroke – Paralysis precipitated by damage to brain cells.

Sulfonylurea – A type of oral medication which helps to reduce the blood sugar level.

Tes-Tape – A type of test strip material used to measure sugar level in urine.

Type 1 Diabetes – Disease characterized by destruction of the pancreatic beta cells which create and secrete insulin.

Type 2 Diabetes – Disease in which the body does not produce enough insulin and/or cannot make efficient use of the insulin it produces.

Vascular – Of or associated with the blood vessels.

Vein – A blood vessel that transports blood to the heart.

Vitrectomy – A type of surgery performed to restore eyesight lost due to vitreous hemorrhage or retinal detachment.

Vitreous – The jellylike transparent tissue of the eyeball behind the lens.

References

The references listed here constitute the source material for much of the information presented in each chapter. They include the suggested readings given at the end of each chapter as well as additional articles from the scholarly and professional literature. Although the latter are intended primarily for health professionals and students, the reader is encouraged to explore those that might shed light on areas of special interest.

To find a reference cited in the text, go directly to the alphabetical master list that follows the chapter-by-chapter citations below. To find supporting data or other background information on subjects covered in a particular chapter, check the chapter listings immediately below. Full reference citations for all sources listed can be found in the master list.

For readings intended specifically for the lay reader, see the section titled "Suggested Reading."

References Listed by Chapter

(full citations in master list below)

Introduction

American Diabetes Association, 1987, 1996a; Bursztajn et al., 1990; Cox & Gonder-Frederick, 1992; Diabetes Control and

Complications Trial Research Group, 1993; Ellis & Harper, 1975; Glasser, 1989; Hamburg et al., 1979; Jacobson, 1996b; Lees, 1983; Lorenz et al., 1996; National Diabetes Data Group, 1995; Pichert, 1983; Raymond, 1992; Rubin et al., 1992; Simon et al., 1995; Sims & Sims, 1992; Surwit et al., 1983; Surwit & Schneider, 1993.

Chapter 1

Hamburg & Inoff, 1983; Hoover, 1979; Koski, 1969; Rubin & Peyrot, 1996; Tonnessen, 1996; Wishner & O'Brien, 1978.

Chapter 2

American Diabetes Association, 1996a, 1998b, 1998c; Beaser & Hill, 1995; Colwell, 1994; Diabetes Control and Complications Trial Research Group, 1993, 1996; Expert Committee on the Diagnosis and Classification of Diabetes Mellitus, 1997; Lebovitz, 1994; Nathan & Laverman, 1997; Pollet & El-Kebbi, 1994; Prashker & Subak-Sharpe, 1995; Ross et al., 1997; Saudek et al., 1997.

Chapter 3

American Diabetes Association, 1997b; Cochran et al., 1979; Diabetes Control and Complications Trial Research Group, 1996; Dunn & Turtle, 1981; Fisher et al., 1982; Fowler et al., 1976; Helz & Templeton, 1990; Hoover, 1979; Klonoff, 1997; Koski, 1969; Lawson et al., 1981; Monagan, 1982; National Diabetes Data Group, 1995; Polonsky, 1996; Rubin et al., 1992; Rubin & Peyrot, 1992; Seeburg & DeBoer, 1980; Simonds, 1977; Sims & Sims, 1992; Surwit & Feinglos, 1983; Surwit & Schneider, 1993; Turkington, 1985.

Chapter 4

American Diabetes Association, 1996a; Cassem, 1979; Crate, 1965; Davis et al., 1965; Frankel, 1975; Hamburg & Inoff, 1983;

Hoover, 1979; Koski, 1969; Kovacs, 1979; Kübler-Ross, 1997; Lustman, 1994; Lustman et al., 1996; Oehler-Giarratana, 1978.

Chapter 5

American Diabetes Association, 1996a, 1996b, 1997a, 1997b; Anderson et al., 1981; Beaser, 1994; Bernstein, 1997; Bursztajn et al., 1990; Cox & Gonder-Frederick, 1992; Diabetes Control and Complications Trial Research Group, 1993; Dinsmoor, 1993; Ellis & Harper, 1975; Glasgow et al., 1997; Glasser, 1989; Helz & Templeton, 1990; Hoover, 1979; Jacobs, 1984; Jacobson, 1996a, 1996b; Jacobson et al., 1994; Klein et al., 1996; Koski & Kumento, 1975; Kovacs et al., 1990b; Lustman, 1994; Marlatt & Gordon, 1985; Nicolucci et al., 1996; Overstreet et al., 1995; Peele et al., 1991; Pennebaker et al., 1981; Polonsky, 1995; Rubin, 1995; Rubin & Peyrot, 1992; Schade et al., 1996; Simon et al., 1995; Steinburg, 1993a, 1993b; Surwit et al., 1983;Valentine et al., 1994; Van der Does et al., 1996.

Chapter 6

Anderson, 1995; Anderson et al., 1995; Anderson et al., 1996; Bursztajn et al., 1990; Charron-Prochownik et al., 1997; Cox & Gonder-Frederick, 1992; Frankel, 1975; Glasgow et al., 1996; Golin et al., 1996; Greenfield et al., 1988, 1995; Groen & Pelser, 1982; Gutheil et al., 1984; Hirsch, 1996; Ho et al., 1997; Hoover, 1979; Jacobson, 1996a; Jacobson & Hauser, 1983; Johnson, 1982; Katz, 1997; Kravitz et al., 1971; Marrero, 1994; Mazzuca et al., 1983; Page et al., 1981; Peters et al., 1996; Pichert et al., 1994; Rost et al., 1991; Solowiejczyk & Baker, 1981; Sullivan, 1978; Surwit et al., 1983; Surwit et al., 1982; Verlato et al., 1996; Weinberger et al., 1984.

Chapter 7

Ahlfield et al., 1983; American Diabetes Association, 1987; Anderson & Auslander, 1980; Anderson et al., 1990; Cederblad et al., 1982; Cox & Gonder-Frederick, 1992; Coyne & Anderson, 1988, 1989; Crain et al., 1966a, 1966b; Grey et al., 1980; Guthrie et al., 1990; Hauser et al., 1990; Hochman, 1984; Jacobson et al., 1994, 1997; Koski et al., 1976; Kovacs et al., 1990a; Marrero et al., 1982; Mattsson, 1979; Minuchin et al., 1975; Minuchin & Barcai, 1969; Overstreet et al., 1995; Rubin et al., 1992; Rubin and Peyrot, 1992; Satin et al., 1989; Surwit & Schneider, 1993; Tarnow & Tomlinson, 1978; Wishner & O'Brien, 1978.

Chapter 8

Anderson & Laffel, 1997; Benedek, 1948; Brink & Moltz, 1997; Drash, 1979; Greydanus & Hofmann, 1979a, 1979b; Hauser et al., 1979; Hoover, 1979; Johnson, 1980; Johnson et al., 1995; Koski et al., 1976; Koski & Kumento, 1975; La Greca, 1991; La Greca et al., 1995; Lawlor et al., 1996; Loring, 1993; Pinhas-Hamiel & Zeitler, 1997; Pond, 1979; Siminerio & Betschart, 1995; Wysocki, 1997.

Chapter 9

Ahlfield et al., 1985; Bartholomew, 1997; Ellis & Harper, 1975; Fisher et al., 1982; Raffel & Rotter, 1986; Task Force for the American Diabetes Association Council on Pregnancy, 1992.

Chapter 10

American Diabetes Association, 1996a, 1998a, 1998d; Baker, 1997; Bell, 1996; Bloomgarden, 1996b; Bursztajn, 1985, 1993; Bursztajn & Brodsky, 1996; Cochran et al., 1979; Dawson, 1995; Edelwich & Brodsky, 1980; Gillespie, 1994; Gilmer et al., 1997; Gordon, 1993; Graham et al., 1995; Greene & Geroy, 1993; Hornsby, 1995; Mathiesen & Borch-Johnsen, 1997; Mawby, 1997; Mazur, 1995; Mohr, 1994; National Diabetes Data Group, 1995; Peters et al., 1996; Quickel, 1994; Rubin, 1982; Rubin et al., 1994; Stoneham, 1995; *Teahan v. Metro-North Commuter R.*

Co., 1996; Thurm & Harper, 1992; *Turco v. Hoechst Celanese Chemical Group Inc.*, 1996.

Chapter 11

Allen et al., 1990; American Diabetes Association, 1996a, 1996c; Benson & Proctor, 1994; Bloomgarden, 1996a; Cox & Gonder-Frederick, 1992; D'Eramo-Melkus et al., 1992; Glasgow et al., 1996; Nathan & Lauerman, 1997; Polonsky et al., 1996; Raffel et al., 1996; Rasch, 1982; Saudek et al., 1997; Smith et al., 1997; Turner & Levy, 1996.

Chapter 12

Anderson et al., 1989; Bernbaum et al., 1989; Blum & Galatzer, 1982; Brink, 1982; Citrin et al., 1982; Edelwich & Brodsky, 1992; Frankel, 1975; Jacobson, 1996b; Oehler-Giarratana & Fitzgerald, 1980; Rubin & Peyrot, 1992; Tattersall et al., 1985; Yalom, 1995.

Master Reference List

Ahlfield, J. E., Soler, N. G., and Marcus, S. D. Adolescent diabetes mellitus: Parent/child perspectives of the effect of the disease on family and social interactions. *Diabetes Care* 6 (1983): 393–398.

Ahlfield, J. E., Soler, N. G., and Marcus, S. D. The young adult with diabetes: Impact of the disease on marriage and having children. *Diabetes Care* 8 (1985): 52–56.

Allen, B. T., DeLong, E. R., and Feussner, J. R. Impact of glucose self-monitoring on non-insulin-treated patients with Type II diabetes mellitus: Randomized controlled trial comparing blood and urine testing. *Diabetes Care* 13 (1990): 1044–1050.

American Diabetes Association. *Diabetes in the Family* (rev. ed.). Alexandria, VA: American Diabetes Association, 1987.

American Diabetes Association. *American Diabetes Association Complete Guide to Diabetes: The Ultimate Home Diabetes Reference*. Alexandria, VA: American Diabetes Association, 1996a (paperback, 1997).

American Diabetes Association. Consensus statement: The pharmacological treatment of hyperglycemia in NIDDM. *Diabetes Care* 19(Suppl. 1) (1996b): 54–61.

American Diabetes Association. Consensus statement: Self-monitoring of blood glucose. *Diabetes Care* 19 (Suppl. 1) (1996c): 62–66.

American Diabetes Association. Position statement: Diabetes mellitus and exercise. *Diabetes Care* 20 (1997a): 1908–1912.

American Diabetes Association. *Type 2 Diabetes: Your Healthy Living Guide* (2nd ed.). Alexandria, VA: American Diabetes Association, 1997b.

American Diabetes Association. Position statement: Hypoglycemia and employment/licensure. *Diabetes Care* 21(Suppl. 1) (1998a): S84.

American Diabetes Association. Position statement: Implications of the Diabetes Control and Complications Trial. *Diabetes Care* 21(Suppl. 1) (1998b): S88–90.

American Diabetes Association. Position statement: Prevention of Type 1 diabetes mellitus. *Diabetes Care* 21(Suppl. 1) (1998c): S83.

American Diabetes Association. Position statement: Third-party reimbursement for diabetes care, self-management education, and supplies. *Diabetes Care* 21(Suppl. 1) (1998d): S86.

American Diabetes Association. *Buyer's Guide to Diabetes Products*. Alexandria, VA: American Diabetes Association [published annually].

Anderson, B. J. and Auslander, W. F. Research on diabetes management and the family: A critique. *Diabetes Care* 3 (1980): 696–702.

Anderson, B. J., Auslander, W. F., Jung, K. C., Miller J. P., and Santiago, J. V. Assessing family sharing of diabetes responsibilities. *Journal of Pediatric Psychology* 15 (1990): 477– 492.

Anderson, B. J. and Laffel, L. M. B. Behavioral and psychosocial research with school-aged children with Type I diabetes. *Diabetes Spectrum* 10 (1997): 277–281.

Anderson, B. J., Miller, J. P., Auslander, W. F., and Santiago, J. V. Family characteristics of diabetic adolescents: Relationship to metabolic control. *Diabetes Care* 4 (1981): 586–594.

Anderson, B. J., Wolf, F. M., Burkhart, M. T., Cornell, R. G., and Bacon, G. E. Effects of peer-group intervention on metabolic control of adolescents with IDDM: Randomized outpatient study. *Diabetes Care* 12 (1989): 179–183.

Anderson, R. M. Patient empowerment and the traditional medical model: A case of irreconcilable differences? *Diabetes Care* 18 (1995): 412–415.

Anderson, R. M., Funnell, M. M., and Arnold, M. S. Using the empowerment approach to help patients change behavior. In B. J. Anderson and R. R. Rubin (Eds.), *Practical Psychology for Diabetes Clinicians*. Alexandria, VA: American Diabetes Association, 1996: 163–172.

Anderson, R. M., Funnell, M. M., Butler, P. M., Arnold, M. S., Fitzgerald, J. T., and Feste, C. C. Patient empowerment: Results of a randomized controlled trial. *Diabetes Care* 18 (1995): 943–949.

Baker, B. Taking it to the states: Insurance reform sweeps the nation as grassroots movements spur state legislators to action. *Diabetes Forecast* May 1997: 44–48.

Bartholomew, S. P. Make way for baby. *Diabetes Forecast* December 1997: 20–33.

Beaser, R. S. *Outsmarting Diabetes: A Dynamic Approach for Reducing the Effects of Insulin-Dependent Diabetes*. Boston, MA: Joslin Diabetes Center, 1994.

Beaser, R. S., with Hill, J. V. C. *The Joslin Guide to Diabetes: A Program for Managing Your Treatment*. New York: Fireside, 1995.

Bell, D. S. H. Alcohol and the NIDDM patient. *Diabetes Care* 19 (1996): 509–513.

References

Benedek T. An approach to the study of the diabetic. *Psychosomatic Medicine* 10 (1948): 284–287.

Benson, H. and Proctor, W. *Beyond the Relaxation Response: How to Harness the Healing Power of Your Personal Beliefs*. New York: Berkley Publishing Group, 1994.

Bernbaum, M., Albert, S. G., Brusca, S. R., Drimmer, A., Duckro, P.N., Cohen, J. D., Trindade, M. C., and Silverberg, A. B. A model clinical program for patients with diabetes and visual impairment. *Diabetes Educator* 15 (1989): 325–330.

Bernstein, R. K. *Dr. Bernstein's Diabetes Solution: A Complete Guide to Achieving Normal Blood Sugars*. Boston: Little, Brown & Co., 1997.

Bloomgarden, Z. T. Conference Report: Approaches to the treatment of Type II diabetes and developments in glucose monitoring and insulin administration. *Diabetes Care* 19 (1996a): 906–909.

Bloomgarden, Z. T. New and traditional treatment of glycemia in NIDDM. *Diabetes Care* 19 (1996b): 295–299.

Blum, A. and Galatzer, A. Group counselling for diabetic patients. *Pediatric and Adolescent Endocrinology* 10 (1982): 230–233.

Brink S. Youth and parents groups for patients with juvenile onset Type I diabetes mellitus. *Pediatric and Adolescent Endocrinology* 10 (1982): 234–240.

Brink, S. J. and Moltz, K. The message of the DCCT for children and adolescents. *Diabetes Spectrum* 10 (1997): 265–267.

Bursztajn, H. J. More law and less protection: 'Critogenesis,' 'legal iatrogenesis,' and medical decision making. *Journal of Geriatric Psychiatry* 18 (1985): 143–153.

Bursztajn, H. J. From PSDA to PTSD: The Patient Self-Determination Act and post-traumatic stress disorder. *Journal of Clinical Ethics* 4 (1993): 71–74.

Bursztajn, H. J. and Brodsky, A. A new resource for managing malpractice risks in managed care. *Archives of Internal Medicine* 156 (1996): 2057–2063.

Bursztajn, H. J., Feinbloom, R. I., Hamm, R. M., and Brodsky, A. *Medical Choices, Medical Chances: How Patients, Families, and Physicians Can Cope with Uncertainty.* New York: Routledge, 1990.

Cassem, N. H. Profiles of coping responses. In B. A. Hamburg, L. F. Lipsett, G. E. Inoff, and A. L. Drash (Eds.). *Behavioral and Psychosocial Issues in Diabetes, Proceedings of the National Conference.* Washington, DC: U.S. Department of Health and Human Services, 1979 (NIH Publication No. 80–1993): 61–64.

Cederblad, M., Helgesson, M., Larsson, Y., and Ludvigsson, J. Family structure and diabetes in children. *Pediatric and Adolescent Endocrinology* 10 (1982): 94–98.

Charron-Prochownik, D., Maihle, T., Siminerio, L., and Songer, T. Outpatient versus inpatient care of children newly diagnosed with IDDM. *Diabetes Care* 20 (1997): 657–660.

Citrin, W. S., Zigo, M. A., LaGreca, A., and Skyler, J. S. Group strategies for diabetes in adolescence. *Pediatric and Adolescent Endocrinology* 10 (1982): 219–223.

Cochran, H. A., Marble, A., and Galloway, J. A. Factors in the survival of patients with insulin-requiring diabetes for 50 years. *Diabetes Care* 2 (1979): 363–368.

Colwell, J. A. DCCT findings: Applicability and implications for NIDDM. *Diabetes Reviews* 2 (1994): 277–291.

Cox, D. J. and Gonder-Frederick, L. Major developments in behavioral diabetes research. *Journal of Consulting and Clinical Psychology* 60 (1992): 628–638.

Coyne, J. C. and Anderson, B. J. The "psychosomatic family" reconsidered: Diabetes in context. *Journal of Marital and Family Therapy* 14 (1988): 113–123.

Coyne, J. C. and Anderson, B. J. The "psychosomatic family" reconsidered II: Recalling a defective model and looking ahead. *Journal of Marital and Family Therapy* 15 (1989): 139–148.

Crain, A. J., Sussman, M. B., and Weil, W. B. Effects of a diabetic child on marital integration and related measures of family functioning. *Journal of Health and Human Behavior* 7 (1966a): 122–127.

Crain, A. J., Sussman, M. B., and Weil, W. B. Family interaction, diabetes, and sibling relationships. *International Journal of Social Psychiatry* 12 (1966b): 35–43.

Crate, M. A. Nursing functions in adaptation to chronic illness. *American Journal of Nursing* 65(10) (1965): 72–76.

Davis, D. M., Schipp, J. C., and Pattishall, E. G. Attitudes of diabetic boys and girls towards diabetes. *Diabetes* 14 (1965): 106–109.

Dawson, L. Y. *Managing Diabetes on a Budget.* Alexandria, VA: American Diabetes Association, 1995.

D'Eramo-Melkus, G. A., Wylie-Rosett, J., and Hagan, J. A. Metabolic impact of education in NIDDM. *Diabetes Care* 15 (1992): 864–869.

Diabetes Control and Complications Trial Research Group. The effect of intensive treatment of diabetes on the development and progression of long-term complications in insulin-dependent diabetes mellitus. *New England Journal of Medicine* 329 (1993): 977–986.

Diabetes Control and Complications Trial Research Group. Influence of intensive diabetes treatment on quality-of-life outcomes in the Diabetes Control and Complications Trial. *Diabetes Care* 19 (1996): 195–203.

Dinsmoor, R. S. How do oral agents work? *Diabetes Self-Management* November/December 1993: 46–49.

Drash, A. L. The child with diabetes mellitus. In B. A. Hamburg, L. F. Lipsett, G. E. Inoff, and A. L. Drash (Eds.). *Behavioral and Psychosocial Issues in Diabetes, Proceedings of the National Conference.* Washington, DC: U.S. Department of Health and Human Services, 1979 (NIH Publication No. 80–1993): 33–42.

Dunn, S. M. and Turtle, J. R. The myth of the diabetic personality. *Diabetes Care* 4 (1981): 640–6.

Edelwich, J. and Brodsky, A. *Burnout: Stages of Disillusionment in the Helping Professions.* New York: Human Sciences Press, 1980.

Edelwich, J. and Brodsky, A. *Group Counseling for the Resistant Client: A Practical Guide to Group Process.* New York: Lexington Books, 1992.

Ellis, A. and Harper, R. A. *A New Guide to Rational Living.* N. Hollywood, CA: Wilshire, 1975.

Expert Committee on the Diagnosis and Classification of Diabetes Mellitus. Report on the diagnosis and classification of diabetes mellitus. *Diabetes Care* 20 (1997): 1183–1197.

References

Fisher, E. B., Delamater, A. M., Bertelson, A. D., and Kirkley, B. G. Psychological factors in diabetes and its treatment. *Journal of Counseling and Clinical Psychology* 50 (1982): 993–1003.

Fowler, J. E., Budzynski, T. H., and Vandenbergh, R. L. Effects of an EMG biofeedback relaxation program on the control of diabetes. *Biofeedback and Self-Regulation* 1 (1976): 105–112.

Frankel, J. J. Juvenile diabetes — the look from within. *Modern Problems in Paediatrics* 12 (1975): 358–360.

Gillespie, S. How to win with your insurance company. *Diabetes Forecast* December 1994: 42–47.

Gilmer, T. P., O'Connor, P. J., Manning, W. G., and Rush, W. A. The cost to health plans of poor glycemic control. *Diabetes Care* 20 (1997): 1847–1853.

Glasgow, R. E., Ruggiero, L., Eakin, E. G., Dryfoos, J., and Chobanian, L. Quality of life and associated characteristics in a large national sample of adults with diabetes. *Diabetes Care* 20 (1997): 562–567.

Glasgow, R. E., Toobert, D. J., and Hampson, S. E. Effects of a brief office-based intervention to facilitate diabetes dietary self-management. *Diabetes Care* 19 (1996): 835–842.

Glasser, W. *Reality Therapy*. New York: HarperCollins, 1989.

Golin, C. E., DiMatteo, M. R., and Gelberg, L. The role of patient participation in the doctor visit: Implications for adherence to diabetes care. *Diabetes Care* 19 (1996): 1153–1164.

Gordon, N. F. *Diabetes: Your Complete Exercise Guide*. Champaign, IL: Human Kinetics Publishers, 1993.

Graham, C., Biermann, J., and Toohey, B. *The Diabetes Sports and Exercise Book: How to Play Your Way to Better Health*. Los Angeles: Lowell House, 1995.

Greene, D. S. and Geroy, G. D. Diabetes and job performance: An empirical investigation. *Diabetes Educator* 19 (1993): 293–298.

Greenfield, S., Kaplan, S. H., Ware J. E., Jr., Yano, E. M., and Frank, H. J. Patients' participation in medical care: Effects on blood sugar control and quality of life in diabetes. *Journal of General Internal Medicine* 3 (1988): 448–457.

Greenfield, S., Rogers, W., Mangotich, M., Carney, M. F., and Tarlov, A. R. Outcomes of patients with hypertension and non-insulin-dependent diabetes mellitus treated by different systems and specialities: Results from the Medical Outcomes Study. *Journal of the American Medical Association* 274 (1995): 1436–1444.

Grey, M. J., Genel, M., and Tamborlane, W. V. Psychosocial adjustment of latency-aged diabetics: determinants and relationship to control. *Pediatrics* 65 (1980): 69–73.

Greydanus, D. E. and Hofmann, A. D. A perspective on the brittle teenage diabetic. *Journal of Family Practice* 9 (1979a): 1007–1012.

Greydanus, D. E. and Hofmann, A. D. Psychological factors in diabetes mellitus: a review of the literature with emphasis on adolescence. *American Journal of Diseases of Children* 133 (1979b): 1061–1066.

Groen, J. J. and Pelser, H. E. Newer concepts of teaching, learning and education and their application to the patient-doctor cooperation in the treatment of diabetes mellitus. *Pediatric and Adolescent Endocrinology* 10 (1982): 168–177.

Gutheil, T. G., Bursztajn, H. J., and Brodsky A. Malpractice prevention through the sharing of uncertainty: informed consent and the therapeutic alliance. *New England Journal of Medicine* 311 (1984): 49–51.

Guthrie, D. W., Sargent, L., Speelman, D., and Parks, L. Effects of parental relaxation training on glycosylated hemoglobin of children with diabetes. *Patient Education and Counseling* 16 (1990): 247–253.

Hamburg, B. A. and Inoff, G. E. Coping with predictable crises of diabetes. *Diabetes Care* 6 (1983): 409–16.

Hamburg, B. A., Lipsett, L. F., Inoff, G. E., and Drash, A. L. (Eds.). *Behavioral and Psychosocial Issues in Diabetes, Proceedings of the National Conference.* Washington, DC: U.S. Department of Health and Human Services, 1979 (NIH Publication No. 80–1993).

Hauser, S. T., Jacobson, A. M., Lavori, P., Wolfsdorf, J. I., Herskowitz, R. D., Milley, J. E., Bliss, R., Wertleib, D., and Stein, J. Adherence among children and adolescents with insulin-dependent diabetes mellitus over a four-year longitudinal follow-up. II. Immediate and long-term linkages with the family milieu. *Journal of Pediatric Psychology* 15 (1990): 527–542.

Hauser, S. T., Pollets, D., Turner, B. L., Jacobson, A., Powers, S., and Noam G. Ego development and self-esteem in diabetic adolescents. *Diabetes Care* 2 (1979): 465–471.

Helz, J. W. and Templeton, B. Evidence of the role of psychosocial factors in diabetes mellitus: A review. *American Journal of Psychiatry* 147 (1990): 1275–1282.

Hirsch, I. B. *How to Get Great Diabetes Care.* Alexandria, VA: American Diabetes Association, 1996.

Ho, M., Marger, M., Beart, J., Yip, I., and Shekelle, P. Is the quality of diabetes care better in a diabetes clinic or in a general medicine clinic? *Diabetes Care* 20 (1997): 472–475.

Hochman, G. Does your family make you sick . . . or well? *American Health* 3(7) (1984): 74–87.

Hoover, J. Another point of view. In B. A. Hamburg, L. F. Lipsett, G. E. Inoff, and A. L. Drash (Eds.). *Behavioral and Psychosocial Issues in Diabetes, Proceedings of the National Conference*. Washington, DC: U.S. Department of Health and Human Services, 1979 (NIH Publication No. 80–1993): 25–32.

Hornsby, W. (Ed.). *The Fitness Book for People with Diabetes: A Project of the American Diabetes Association Council on Exercise*. Alexandria, VA: American Diabetes Association, 1995.

Jacobs, S. V. Stress and the course of insulin-dependent diabetes mellitus: a psychosocial and physiological investigation. Doctoral dissertation, Harvard University, Department of Psychology and Social Relations, 1984.

Jacobson, A. M. Improving glycemic control in patients with Type I diabetes. In B. J. Anderson and R. R. Rubin (Eds.), *Practical Psychology for Diabetes Clinicians*. Alexandria, VA: American Diabetes Association, 1996a: 105–112.

Jacobson, A. M. The psychological care of patients with insulin-dependent diabetes mellitus. *New England Journal of Medicine* 334 (1996b): 1249–1253.

Jacobson, A. M. and Hauser, S. T. Behavioral and psychological aspects of diabetes. In M. Ellenberg and H. Rifkin (Eds.). *Diabetes Mellitus: Theory and Practice* (3rd ed.). New Hyde Park, NY: Medical Examination Publishing Co., 1983: 1037–52.

Jacobson, A. M., Hauser, S. T., Lavori, P., Willett, J. B., Cole, C. F., Wolfsdorf, J. I., Dumont, R. H., and Wertleib, D. Family environment and glycemic control: A four-year prospective study of children and adolescents with insulin-dependent diabetes mellitus. *Psychosomatic Medicine* 56 (1994): 401–409.

Jacobson, A. M., Hauser, S. T., Willett, J. B., Wolfsdorf, J. I., Dvorak, R., Herman, L., and de Groot, M. Psychological adjustment to IDDM: 10-year follow-up of an onset cohort of child and adolescent patients. *Diabetes Care* 20 (1997): 811–818.

Johnson, J. B. Diabetes education: it is not only what we say. *Diabetes Care* 5 (1982): 343–345.

Johnson, R. W., Johnson, S., Kleinman, U., and Johnson, R. *Managing Your Child's Diabetes* (rev. ed.). New York: MasterMedia Ltd., 1995.

Johnson, S. B. Psychosocial factors in juvenile diabetes: a review. *Journal of Behavioral Medicine* 3 (1980): 95–116.

Katz, J. *The Silent World of Doctor and Patient.* Baltimore: Johns Hopkins University Press, 1997.

Klein, R., Klein, B. E. K., Moss, S. E., and Cruickshanks, K. J. The medical management of hyperglycemia over a 10-year period in people with diabetes. *Diabetes Care* 19 (1996): 744–750.

Klonoff, D. C. Noninvasive blood glucose monitoring. *Diabetes Care* 20 (1997): 433– 437.

Koski, M. L. The coping process in childhood diabetes. *Acta Paediatrica Scandinavica* 198(Suppl.) (1969): 1–56.

Koski, M. L., Ahlas, A., and Kumento, A. A psychosomatic follow-up study of childhood diabetics. *Acta Paedopsychiatrica* 42 (1976): 12–26.

Koski, M. L., and Kumento, A. Adolescent development and behavior: a psychosomatic follow-up study of childhood diabetics. *Modern Problems in Paediatrics* 12 (1975): 348–353.

Kovacs, M. Depression and 'adaptation' in juvenile diabetics. In B. A. Hamburg, L. F. Lipsett, G. E. Inoff, and A. L. Drash (Eds.). *Behavioral and Psychosocial Issues in Diabetes, Proceedings of the National Conference.* Washington, DC: U.S. Department of Health and Human Services, 1979 (NIH Publication No. 80–1993): 57–60.

Kovacs, M., Iyengar, S., Goldston, D., Obrosky, D. S., Stewart, J., and Marsh, J. Psychological functioning among mothers of children with insulin-dependent diabetes mellitus: A longitudinal study. *Journal of Consulting and Clinical Psychology* 58 (1990a): 189–195.

Kovacs, M., Iyengar, A., Goldston, D., Stewart, J., Obrosky, D. S., and Marsh, J. Psychological functioning of children with insulin-dependent diabetes mellitus: A longitudinal study. *Journal of Pediatric Psychology* 15 (1990b): 619–632.

Kravitz, A. R., Isenberg, P. L., Shore, M. F., and Barnett, D. M. Emotional factors in diabetes mellitus. In A. Marble, P. White, R. F. Bradley, and L. P. Krall (Eds.). *Joslin's Diabetes Mellitus* (11th ed.). Philadelphia: Lea & Febiger, 1971: 767–82.

Kübler-Ross, E. *On Death and Dying.* New York: Collier Books, 1997.

La Greca, A. M. Commentary. *Diabetes Spectrum* 4 (1991): 269–271.

La Greca, A. M., Auslander, W. F., Greco, P., Spetter, D., Fisher, E. B., and Santiago, J. V. I get by with a little help from my family and friends: Adolescents' support for diabetes care. *Journal of Pediatric Psychology* 20 (1995): 449–476.

Lawlor, M. T., Laffel, L. M. B., Anderson, B. J., and Bertorelli, A. *Caring for Young Children Living with Diabetes: A Manual for Parents.* Boston, MA: Joslin Diabetes Center, 1996.

Lawson, V. K., Young, R. T., Kitabchi, A. E. Maturity-onset diabetes of the young: an illustrative case for control of diabetes and hormonal normalization with dietary management. *Diabetes Care* 4 (1981): 108–112.

Lebovitz, H. E. The DCCT and its implications for NIDDM. *Clinical Diabetes* January/February 1994: 3–4.

Lees, M. More on reactions . . . *Pumpers* January 1983: 1, 8.

Lorenz, R. A., Bubb, J., Davis, D., Jacobson, A., Jannasch, K., Kramer, J., Lipps, J., and Schlundt, D. Changing behavior: Practical lessons from the Diabetes Control and Complications Trial. *Diabetes Care* 19 (1996): 648–652.

Loring, G. *Parenting a Diabetic Child: A Practical, Empathetic Guide to Help You and Your Child Live with Diabetes.* Los Angeles: Lowell House, 1993.

Lustman, P. J. (Ed.). Depression in adults with diabetes. *Diabetes Spectrum* 7 (1994): 161–189.

Lustman, P. J., Griffith, L. S., and Clouse, R. E. Recognizing and managing depression in patients with diabetes. In B. J. Anderson and R. R. Rubin (Eds.). *Practical Psychology for Diabetes Clinicians.* Alexandria, VA: American Diabetes Association, 1996: 143–154.

Marlatt, G. A. and Gordon, J. R. *Relapse Prevention: Maintenance Strategies in the Treatment of Addictive Behaviors.* New York: Guilford, 1985.

Marrero, D. G. Current effectiveness of diabetes health care in the U.S.: How far from the ideal? *Diabetes Reviews* 2 (1994): 292–309.

Marrero, D. G., Lau, N., Golden, M. P., Kershnar, A., and Myers, G. C. Family dynamics in adolescent diabetes mellitus: parental behavior and metabolic control. *Pediatric and Adolescent Endocrinology* 10 (1982): 77–82.

Mathiesen, B. and Borch-Johnsen, K. Diabetes and accident insurance: A three-year follow-up of 7,599 insured diabetic individuals. *Diabetes Care* 20 (1997): 1781–1784.

Mattsson, A. Juvenile diabetes: impacts on life stages and systems. In B. A. Hamburg, L. F. Lipsett, G. E. Inoff, and A. L. Drash (Eds.). *Behavioral and Psychosocial Issues in Diabetes, Proceedings of the National Conference.* Washington, DC: U.S. Department of Health and Human Services, 1979 (NIH Publication No. 80–1993): 43–55.

Mawby, M. Time for law to catch up with life. *Diabetes Care* 20 (1997): 1640–1641.

Mazur, M. L. Fighting back. *Diabetes Forecast* August 1995: 16–22.

Mazzuca, S. A., Weinberger, M., Kurpius, D. J., Froehle, T. C., and Heister, M. Clinician communication associated with diabetic patients' comprehension of their therapeutic regimen. *Diabetes Care* 6 (1983): 347–350.

Minuchin, S., Baker, L., Rosman, B. L., Liebman, R., Milman, L., and Todd, T. C. A conceptual model of psychosomatic illness in children. *Archives of General Psychiatry* 32 (1975): 1031–1038.

Minuchin, S. and Barcai, A. Therapeutically induced family crisis. In J. H. Masserman (Ed.). *Science and Psychoanalysis* (Vol. 14): *Childhood and Adolescence.* New York: Grune & Stratton, 1969: 199–205.

Mohr, M. Have you heard about COBRA? *Diabetes Forecast* December 1994: 63.

Monagan, D. One man's triumph over diabetes. *America's Health* 4 (2) (1982): 10–13.

Nathan, D. M., with Lauerman, J. F. *Diabetes: The Most Comprehensive, Up-to-Date Information Available to Help You Understand Your Condition, Make the Right Treatment Choices, and Cope Effectively (A Massachusetts General Hospital Book)*. New York: Times Books, 1997.

National Diabetes Data Group. *Diabetes in America* (2nd ed.) (NIH Publication No. 95–1468). Bethesda, MD: National Institutes of Health, National Institute of Diabetes and Digestive and Kidney Diseases, 1995.

Nicolucci, A., Cavaliere, D., Scorpiglione, N., Carinci, F., Capani, F., Tognoni, G., and Benedetti, M. M. A comprehensive assessment of the avoidability of long-term complications of diabetes: A case-control study. *Diabetes Care* 19 (1996): 927–933.

Oehler-Giarratana, J. Meeting the challenge. *Diabetes Forecast* 31(2) (1978): 31–33.

Oehler-Giarratana, J. and Fitzgerald, R. G. Group therapy with blind diabetics. *Archives of General Psychiatry* 37 (1980): 463–467.

Overstreet, S., Goins, J., Chen, R. S., Holmes, C. S., Greer, T., Dunlap, W. P., and Frentz J. Family environment and the interrelation of family structure, child behavior, and metabolic control for children with diabetes. *Journal of Pediatric Psychology* 20 (1995): 435–447.

Page, P., Verstracte, D. G., Robb, J. R., and Etzwiler, D. D. Patient recall of self-care recommendations in diabetes. *Diabetes Care* 4 (1981): 96–98.

Peele, S., Brodsky, A., and Arnold, M. *The Truth about Addiction and Recovery: The Life Process Program for Outgrowing Destructive Habits.* New York: Simon and Schuster, 1991.

Pennebaker, J. W., Cox, D. J., Gonder-Frederick, L., Wunsch, M. G., Evans, W. S., and Pohl, S. Physical symptoms related to blood glucose in insulin-dependent diabetics. *Psychosomatic Medicine* 6 (1981): 489–500.

Peters, A. L., Legorreta, A. P., Ossorio, R. C., and Davidson, M. B. Quality of outpatient care provided to diabetic patients: A health maintenance organization experience. *Diabetes Care* 19 (1996): 601–606.

Pichert, J. W. Diabetes in the national TV news: 1971–1981. *Diabetes Care* 6 (1983): 92–94.

Pichert, J. W., Smeltzer, C., Snyder, G. M., Gregory, R. P., Smeltzer R., and Kinzer, C. K. Traditional vs. anchored instruction for diabetes-related nutritional knowledge, skills, and behavior. *Diabetes Educator* 20 (1994): 45–48.

Pinhas-Hamiel, O. and Zeitler, P. A weighty problem – diagnosis and treatment of type 2 diabetes in adolescents. *Diabetes Spectrum* 10 (1997): 292–297.

Pollet, R. J. and El-Kebbi, I. M. The applicability and implications of the DCCT to NIDDM. *Diabetes Reviews* 2 (1994): 413–427.

Polonsky, K. S., Sturis, J., and Bell, G. I. Non-insulin-dependent diabetes mellitus – a genetically programmed failure of the beta cell to compensate for insulin resistance. *New England Journal of Medicine* 334 (1996): 777–783.

Polonsky, W. H. Besieged by the diabetes police. *Diabetes Self-Management* July–August 1995: 21–26.

Polonsky, W. H. Understanding and treating patients with diabetes burnout. In B. J. Anderson and R. R. Rubin (Eds.). *Practical Psychology for Diabetes Clinicians*. Alexandria, VA: American Diabetes Association, 1996: 183–192.

Pond, H. Parental attitudes toward children with a chronic medical disorder: special reference to diabetes mellitus. *Diabetes Care* 2 (1979): 425–431.

Prashker, B. A. and Subak-Sharpe, G. J. (Eds.). *The Columbia University College of Physicians and Surgeons Complete Home Medical Guide* (3rd ed.). New York: Crown, 1995.

Quickel, K. E. Managed health care and intensified management of diabetes. *Diabetes Reviews* 2 (1994): 403–412.

Raffel, L. J., Robbins, D. C., Norris, J. M., Boerwinkle, E., DeFronzo, R. A., Elbein, S. C., Fujimoto, W., Hanis, C. L., Kahn, S. E., Permutt, M. A., Chiu, K. C., Cruz, J., Ehrmann, D. A., Robertson, R. P., Rotter, J. I., and Buse J. The GENNID Study. *Diabetes Care* 19 (1996): 864–872.

Raffel, L. J. and Rotter, J. I. Genetic counseling for families of persons with diabetes mellitus. *Medical Aspects of Human Sexuality* 20(2) (1986): 51–54.

Rasch, L. Controlling glucose in diabetes: must we hit the bullseye? *Therapaeia* September 29 1982: 31–39.

Raymond, M. *The Human Side of Diabetes: Beyond Doctors, Diets, and Drugs*. Chicago: Noble Press, 1992.

Ross, C., Langer, R. D., and Barrett-Connor, E. Given diabetes, is fat better than thin? *Diabetes Care* 20 (1997): 650–652.

Rost, K. M., Flavin, K. S., Cole, K., and McGill, J. B. Change in metabolic control and functional status after hospitalization: Impact of patient activation intervention in diabetic patients. *Diabetes Care* 14 (1991): 881–889.

Rubin, R. J., Altman, W. M., and Mendelson, D. N. Special article: Health care expenditure for people with diabetes mellitus, 1992. *Journal of Clinical Endocrinology and Metabolism* 78 (1994): 809A–809F.

Rubin R. R. Rising to the challenge of tight control. *Diabetes Self-Management* January/February 1995: 6–10.

Rubin, R. R., Biermann, J., and Toohey, B. *Psyching Out Diabetes: A Positive Approach to Your Negative Emotions.* Los Angeles: Lowell House, 1992.

Rubin, R. R. and Peyrot, M. Psychosocial problems and interventions in diabetes: A review of the literature. *Diabetes Care* 15 (1992): 1640–1657.

Rubin, R. R. and Peyrot, M. Emotional responses to diagnosis. In B. J. Anderson and R. R. Rubin (Eds.). *Practical Psychology for Diabetes Clinicians.* Alexandria, VA: American Diabetes Association, 1996: 155–162.

Rubin, W. Treatment for diabetes: a modern medical tragedy? *Family Practice News* 12(6) (1982): 1, 69–81.

Satin, W., La Greca, A. M., Zigo, M. A., and Skyler, J. S. Diabetes in adolescence: Effects of multifamily group intervention and parent simulation of diabetes. *Journal of Pediatric Psychology* 14 (1989): 259–275.

Saudek, C. D., Rubin, R. R., and Shump, C. S. *The Johns Hopkins Guide to Diabetes: For Today and Tomorrow (Johns Hopkins Health Book).* Baltimore: Johns Hopkins University Press, 1997.

Schade, D. S., Boyle, P. J., and Burge, M. R. (Eds.). *101 Tips for Staying Healthy with Diabetes (& Avoiding Complications): A Project of the American Diabetes Association*. Alexandria, VA: American Diabetes Association, 1996.

Seeburg, K. N. and DeBoer, K. F. Effects of EMG biofeedback on diabetes. *Biofeedback and Self-Regulation* 5 (1980): 289–293.

Siminerio, L. and Betschart, J. E. *Raising a Child with Diabetes*. Alexandria, VA: American Diabetes Association, 1995.

Simon, S. B., Howe, L. W., and Kirschenbaum, H. *Values Clarification: The Classic Guide to Discovering Your Truest Feelings, Beliefs, and Goals*. New York: Warner Books, 1995.

Simonds, J. F. Psychiatric status of diabetic youth matched with a control group. *Diabetes* 26 (1977): 921–925.

Sims, D. F. and Sims, E. A. H. (Eds.). *The Other Diabetes: Your Guide to Living with Non-Insulin-Dependent (Type II) Diabetes* (rev. ed.). Alexandria, VA: American Diabetes Association, 1992.

Skyler, J. S. Psychological issues in diabetes. *Diabetes Care* 4 (1981): 656–657.

Smith, D. E., Heckemeyer, C. M., Kratt, P. P., and Mason, D. A. Motivational interviewing to improve adherence to a behavioral weight-control program for older obese women with NIDDM: A pilot study. *Diabetes Care* 20 (1997): 52–54.

Solowiejczyk, J. N. and Baker, L. Physician-patient communication in chronic illness. *Diabetes Care* 4 (1981): 427–429.

Steinburg, C. So what *is* tight control? *Diabetes Forecast* September 1993a: 55–58.

Steinburg, C. Tight for type II, too? *Diabetes Forecast* September 1993b: 61–62.

Stoneham, L. Health insurance: more options, more opportunities: educating companies to cover test strips, preventive care. *Real Living with Diabetes* March–April 1995: 6–8.

Sullivan, B. J. Self-esteem and depression in adolescent diabetic girls. *Diabetes Care* 1 (1978): 18–22.

Surwit, R. S. and Feinglos, M. N. The effects of relaxation on glucose tolerance in non-insulin-dependent diabetes. *Diabetes Care* 6 (1983): 176–179.

Surwit, R. S., Feinglos, M. N., and Scovern, A. W. Diabetes and behavior: a paradigm for health psychology. *American Psychologist* 38 (1983): 255–262.

Surwit, R. S. and Schneider, M. S. Role of stress in the etiology and treatment of diabetes mellitus. *Psychosomatic Medicine* 55 (1993): 380–393.

Surwit, R. S., Scovern, A. W., and Feinglos, M. N. The role of behavior in diabetes care. *Diabetes Care* 5 (1982): 337–342.

Tarnow, J. D. and Tomlinson, N. Juvenile diabetes: impact on the child and family. *Psychosomatics* 19 (1978): 487–491.

Task Force for the American Diabetes Association Council on Pregnancy. *Diabetes and Pregnancy: What to Expect.* Alexandria, VA: American Diabetes Association, 1992.

Tattersall, R. B., McCulloch, D. K., and Aveline, M. Group therapy in the treatment of diabetes. *Diabetes Care* 8 (1985): 180–188.

Teahan v. Metro-North Commuter R. Co., 80 F. 3d 50 (2nd Cir. 1996).

References

Thurm, U. and Harper, P. N. I'm running on insulin: Summary of the history of the International Diabetic Athletes Association. *Diabetes Care* 15 (Suppl. 4) (1992): 1811–1813.

Tonnessen, D. *50 Essential Things to Do When the Doctor Says It's Diabetes*. New York: Plume, 1996.

Turco v. Hoechst Celanese Chemical Group, Inc., 101 F. 3d 1090 (5th Cir. 1996).

Turkington, C. Stress found to play major role in onset, treatment of diabetes. *APA Monitor* February 1985: 28, 37.

Turner, R. C. and Levy, J. C. Notes on the GENNID Study. *Diabetes Care* 19 (1996): 892–895.

Valentine, V., Biermann, J., and Toohey, B. *Diabetes Type II and What to Do*. Los Angeles: Lowell House, 1994.

Van der Does, F. E. E., De Neeling, J. N. D., Snoek, F. J., Kostense, P. J., Grootenhuis, P. A., Bouter, L. M., and Heine, R. J. Symptoms and well-being in relation to glycemic control in type II diabetes. *Diabetes Care* 19 (1996): 204–210.

Verlato, G., Muggeo, M., Bonora, E., Corbellini, M., Bressan, F., and de Marco, R. Attending the diabetes center is associated with increased 5-year survival probability of diabetic patients: The Verona Diabetes Study. *Diabetes Care* 19 (1996): 211–213.

Weinberger, M., Cohen, S. J., and Mazzuca, S. A. The role of physicians' knowledge and attitudes in effective diabetes management. *Social Science and Medicine* 19 (1984): 965–969.

Wishner, W. J. and O'Brien, M. D. Diabetes and the family. *Medical Clinics of North America* 62 (1978): 849–856.

Wysocki, T. *The Ten Keys to Helping Your Child Grow Up with Diabetes: A Practical Guide for Parents & Caregivers*. Alexandria, VA: American Diabetes Association, 1997.

Yalom, I. D. *The Theory and Practice of Group Psychotherapy* (4th ed.). New York: Basic Books, 1995.

References

Suggested Reading

For Persons with Diabetes and Their Families (also useful for health professionals)

Diabetes (general self-help books)

American Diabetes Association. *American Diabetes Association Complete Guide to Diabetes: The Ultimate Home Diabetes Reference*. Alexandria, VA: American Diabetes Association, 1996 (paperback, 1997).

American Diabetes Association. *Diabetes A to Z* (3rd ed.). Alexandria, VA: American Diabetes Association, 1997.

American Diabetes Association. *Diabetes in the Family* (rev. ed.). Alexandria, VA: American Diabetes Association, 1987.

Anderson, J. W. *Diabetes: A Practical New Guide to Healthy Living*. NewYork: Warner Books, 1995.

Beaser, R. S. with Hill, J. V. C. *The Joslin Guide to Diabetes: A Program for Managing Your Treatment*. New York: Fireside, 1995.

Bernstein, R. K. *Dr. Bernstein's Diabetes Solution: A Complete Guide to Achieving Normal Blood Sugars*. Boston: Little Brown, 1997.

Biermann, J. and Toohey, B. *The Diabetic's Book: All Your Questions Answered*. New York: Tarcher, 1994.

Biermann, J. and Toohey, B. *The Diabetic's Total Health Book*. Los Angeles: Tarcher, 1992.

Hirsch, I. B. *How to Get Great Diabetes Care*. Alexandria, VA: American Diabetes Association, 1997.

Joslin Diabetes Center. *Joslin's Diabetes Series* (packet of 6 booklets). Boston: Joslin Diabetes Center, 1992/1998.

Jovanovic-Peterson, L., Biermann, J., and Toohey, B. *The Diabetic Woman* (rev. ed.). New York: Tarcher/Putnam, 1996.

Juliano, J. *When Diabetes Complicates Your Life: Controlling Diabetes and Related Complications* (2nd rev. ed.). Minneapolis: Chronimed, 1998.

Nathan, D. M. with Lauerman, J. F. *Diabetes: The Most Comprehensive, Up-to-Date Information Available to Help You Understand Your Condition, Make the Right Treatment Choices, and Cope Effectively (A Massachusetts General Hospital Book)*. New York: Times Books, 1997.

Pfeifer, M. *Dear Diabetes Advisor*. Alexandria, VA: American Diabetes Association, 1997.

Saudek, C. D., Rubin, R. R., and Shump, C. S. *The Johns Hopkins Guide to Diabetes: For Today and Tomorrow (Johns Hopkins Health Book)*. Baltimore: Johns Hopkins University Press, 1997.

Suggested Reading

Schade, D. S., Boyle, P. J., and Burge, M. R. (Eds.). *101 Tips for Improving Your Blood Sugar.* Alexandria, VA: American Diabetes Association, 1995.

Schade, D. S., Boyle, P. J., and Burge, M. R. (Eds.). *101 Tips for Staying Healthy With Diabetes (& Avoiding Complications).* Alexandria, VA: American Diabetes Association, 1996.

Tonnessen, D. *50 Essential Things to Do When the Doctor Says It's Diabetes.* New York: Plume, 1996.

Type 1

American Diabetes Association. *Right from the Start, Type 1 Diabetes.* Alexandria, VA: American Diabetes Association, 1998.

American Diabetes Association. *The Take-Charge Guide to Type I Diabetes.* Alexandria, VA: American Diabetes Association, 1994.

Beaser, R. S. *Outsmarting Diabetes: A Dynamic Approach for Reducing the Effects of Insulin-Dependent Diabetes.* Boston: Joslin Diabetes Center, 1994.

Type 2

American Diabetes Association. *Right from the Start, Type 2 Diabetes.* Alexandria, VA: American Diabetes Association, 1998.

American Diabetes Association. *Type 2 Diabetes: Your Healthy Living Guide* (2nd ed.). Alexandria, VA: American Diabetes Association, 1997.

Jovanovic-Peterson, L. and Peterson, C. M. *A Touch of Diabetes* (revised and expanded). Minneapolis: Chronimed, 1995.

Valentine, V., Biermann, J., and Toohey, B. *Diabetes Type II and What to Do*. Los Angeles: Lowell House, 1994.

Medical Decision Making and Practical and Emotional Self-Help

Benson, H. and Proctor, W. *Beyond the Relaxation Response: How to Harness the Healing Power of Your Personal Beliefs*. New York: Berkley Publishing Group, 1994.

Bursztajn, H. J., Feinbloom, R. I., Hamm, R. M., and Brodsky, A. *Medical Choices, Medical Chances: How Patients, Families, and Physicians Can Cope with Uncertainty*. New York: Routledge, 1990.

Ellis, A. and Harper, R. A. *A New Guide to Rational Living*. N. Hollywood, CA: Wilshire, 1975.

Glasser, W. *Reality Therapy*. New York: HarperCollins, 1989.

Kelley, D. B. *Caring for the Diabetic Soul: Restoring Emotional Balance for Yourself and Your Family*. Alexandria, VA: American Diabetes Association, 1997.

Peele, S., Brodsky, A., and Arnold, M. *The Truth about Addiction and Recovery: The Life Process Program for Outgrowing Destructive Habits*. New York: Simon and Schuster, 1991.

Raymond, M. *The Human Side of Diabetes: Beyond Doctors, Diets, and Drugs*. Chicago: Noble Press, 1992.

Rubin, R. R., Biermann, J., and Toohey, B. *Psyching Out Diabetes: A Positive Approach to Your Negative Emotions*. Los Angeles: Lowell House, 1992.

Simon, S. B., Howe, L. W., and Kirschenbaum, H. *Values Clarification: The Classic Guide to Discovering Your Truest Feelings, Beliefs, and Goals.* New York: Warner Books, 1995.

For Parents

Hollerorth, Hugo J. *A Guide for Parents of Children and Youth with Diabetes.* Boston: Joslin Diabetes Center, 1994.

Johnson, R. W., Johnson, S., Kleinman, U., and Johnson, R. *Managing Your Child's Diabetes* (rev. ed.). New York: MasterMedia Ltd., 1995.

Lawlor, M. T., Laffel, L. M. B., Anderson, B.J., and Bertorelli, A. *Caring for Young Children Living with Diabetes: A Manual for Parents.* Boston: Joslin Diabetes Center, 1996.

Loring, G. *Parenting a Diabetic Child: A Practical, Empathetic Guide to Help You and Your Child Live with Diabetes.* Los Angeles: Lowell House, 1993.

Siminerio, L. and Betschart, J. E. *Raising a Child with Diabetes.* Alexandria, VA: American Diabetes Association, 1995.

Wysocki, T. *The Ten Keys to Helping Your Child Grow Up with Diabetes: A Practical Guide for Parents & Caregivers.* Alexandria, VA: American Diabetes Association, 1997.

Cooking and Nutrition

American Diabetes Association. *The American Diabetes Association/The American Dietetic Association Family Cookbook: The American Tradition.* New York: Simon & Schuster, 1991.

Better Homes and Gardens Diabetic Cookbook. Des Moines, IA: Better Homes & Gardens, 1992.

Chantiles, V. L. *Diabetic Cooking from Around the World*. New York: Crescent Books, 1995.

Finsand, M. J. *The Complete Diabetic Cookbook*. New York: Sterling Publications, 1990.

Hell, M. A. and Tougas, J. G. *The Art of Cooking for the Diabetic*. New York: Contemporary Books, 1996.

Polin, B. S. and Giedt, F. T. *The Joslin Diabetes Gourmet Cookbook: Heart-Healthy, Everyday Recipes for Family and Friends*. New York: Bantam, 1994.

Soneral, L. M. *The Type II Diabetes Cookbook: Simple and Delicious Low-Sugar, Low-Fat, and Low-Cholesterol Recipes*. Los Angeles: Lowell House, 1997.

Webb, R. *Diabetic Meals in 30 Minutes – Or Less!* Alexandria, VA: American Diabetes Association, 1996.

Sports and Exercise

Gordon, N. F. *Diabetes: Your Complete Exercise Guide*. Champaign, IL: Human Kinetics Publishers, 1993.

Graham, C., Biermann, J., and Toohey, B. *The Diabetes Sports and Exercise Book: How to Play Your Way to Better Health*. Los Angeles: Lowell House, 1995.

Hornsby, W. (Ed.). *The Fitness Book for People with Diabetes: A Project of the American Diabetes Association Council on Exercise*. Alexandria, VA: American Diabetes Association, 1995.

Budgeting and Cost-Cutting

American Diabetes Association. *Buyer's Guide to Diabetes Products*. Alexandria, VA: American Diabetes Association [published annually].

Dawson, L. Y. *Managing Diabetes on a Budget*. Alexandria, VA: American Diabetes Association, 1995.

Personal Commentaries

Bradley, D. J. *Sweet Recovery: A Young Woman's Emotional Ride With Diabetes, Vision Loss, and an Eating Disorder . . . to Health and Freedom*. Upbeat Productions, 1992.

Hightower, G. P. *Sweet Pea: The Autobiography of a Diabetic*. Christopher Publishing House, 1994.

For Health Professionals

Alberti, K. G. M. M., DeFronzo, R. A., Keen, H., and Zimmet, P. *International Textbook of Diabetes Mellitus* (2 vol.). Chichester, U.K.: Wiley, 1992.

American Diabetes Association. (Eds.). *Economic Consequences of Diabetes Mellitus in the U.S. in 1997*. Alexandria, VA: American Diabetes Association, 1998.

Anderson, B. J. and Rubin, R. R. *Practical Psychology for Diabetes Clinicians: How to Deal with the Key Behavioral Issues Faced by Patients and Health-Care Teams*. Alexandria, VA: American Diabetes Association, 1996.

Brown, F. M. and Hare, J. W. *Diabetes Complicating Pregnancy: The Joslin Clinic Method*. New York: Wiley-Liss, 1995.

Brownlee, M. and King, G. L. (Eds.). Chronic complications of diabetes. *Endocrinology and Metabolism Clinics of North America 25* (1996): 217–490.

Campaigne, B. N. and Lampman, R. M. *Exercise in the Clinical Management of Diabetes*. Champaign, IL: Human Kinetics, 1994.

DeFronzo, R. A. *Current Therapy of Diabetes Mellitus*. St. Louis: Mosby, 1998.

Edelwich, J. and Brodsky, A. *Group Counseling for the Resistant Client: A Practical Guide to Group Process*. New York: Lexington Books, 1992.

Finucane, P., Sinclair, A. J., and Finucane, F. (Eds.). *Diabetes in Old Age*. New York: Wiley, 1995.

Haire-Joshu, D. *Management of Diabetes Mellitus: Perspectives of Care Across the Life Span* (2nd ed.). St. Louis: Mosby, 1996.

Hirsch, I. B. and Riddle, M. C. (Eds.). Current therapies for diabetes. *Endocrinology and Metabolism Clinics of North America 26* (1997): 443–701.

Holmes, C. S. (Ed.). *Neuropsychological and Behavioral Aspects of Insulin- and Non-Insulin-Dependent Diabetes*. New York: Springer-Verlag, 1990.

Kahn, C. and Weir, G. (Eds.). *Joslin's Diabetes Mellitus* (13th ed.). Philadelphia: Lea & Febiger, 1994.

Kelnar, C. J. H. (Ed.). *Childhood and Adolescent Diabetes*. London: Chapman & Hall Medical, 1995.

Kongstvedt, P. R. *The Managed Health Care Handbook* (3rd ed.). Gaithersburg, MD: Aspen, 1996.

Lawlor, M. T., Laffel, L. M. B., Anderson, B. J., and Bertorelli, A. *Caring for Young Children Living with Diabetes: A Manual for Health-Care Professionals.* Boston: Joslin Diabetes Center, 1996.

LeRoith, D., Taylor, S. I., and Olefsky, J. M. (Eds.). *Diabetes Mellitus: A Fundamental and Clinical Text.* Philadelphia: Lippincott-Raven, 1996.

National Diabetes Data Group. *Diabetes in America* (2nd ed.) (NIH Publication No. 95–1468). Bethesda, MD: National Institutes of Health, National Institute of Diabetes and Digestive and Kidney Diseases, 1995.

Pickup, J. C. and Williams, G. (Eds.). *Chronic Complications of Diabetes.* Oxford, U.K.: Blackwell Scientific Publications, 1994.

Porte, D., Jr. and Sherwin, R. S. (Eds.). *Ellenberg & Rifkin's Diabetes Mellitus* (5th ed.). Stamford, CT: Appleton & Lange, 1997.

Useful Resources

For additional listings of organizations (including state ADA affiliates), publications, and educational materials, see the *American Diabetes Association Complete Guide to Diabetes* (cited in Suggested Readings), the *Complete Directory for People with Chronic Illness* (Lakeville, CT: Grey House Publishing, 1998/99 and later editions), and the online sources listed below.

On the World Wide Web

Because Internet addresses are subject to change, the surest route to online information about diabetes is to start with a stable organization such as the American Diabetes Association and then find links to other web sites. "Maverick" web sites may be best located by using a search engine or by learning about them through informal channels.

Some of the websites listed here maintain online newsletters or discussion groups or offer links to such resources on other sites.

ABLEDATA
(Information on assistive technology and rehabilitation equipment)
http://www.abledata.com

American Association of Diabetes Educators
http: //www.AADEnet.org

American Diabetes Association
http: //www.diabetes.org

American Foundation for the Blind
http://www.afb.org/afb

American Heart Association
http://www.amhrt.org

Americans with Disabilities Act Technical Assistance Centers
U.S. Department of Justice
http://www.usdoj.gov
http://www.adaptenv.org

Center for Disease Control & Prevention Diabetes Home Page
http: //www.cdc.gov/nccdphp/ddt/ddthome.htm

Children With Diabetes
http: //www.castleweb.com/diabetes/index.html

Combined Health Information Database
http: //chid.nih.gov/subfile/contribs/dm.html

The Diabetes Center
http: //diabetes.sciweb.com

Diabetes Interview [newsletter]
http: //www.diabetesworld.com

Equal Employment Opportunity Commission
http://www.eeoc.gov

Family Voices
http://www.familyvoices.org

Federation for Children with Special Needs
http://www.fcsn.org

Forensic Psychiatry and Medicine
(Americans with Disabilities Act, managed care, insurance, and other medical-legal and mental health issues)
http: //www.forensic-psych.com

Health Insurance Association of America
http://www.hiaa.org

International Diabetic Athletes Association
http://www.getnet.com/~idaa/

Job Accommodation Network
http://janweb.icdi.wvu.edu

Joslin Diabetes Center
http: //www.joslin.harvard.edu

Juvenile Diabetes Foundation International
http: //www.jdfcure.com

National Diabetes Information Clearinghouse
http: //www.niddk.nih.gov

National Federation of the Blind
http://www.nfb.org

National Kidney Foundation
http://www.mcw.edu/nkf

National Rehabilitation Information Center (NARIC)
http://www.naric.com/naric

Recordings for the Blind and Dyslexic
http://www.rfbd.org

Useful Resources

Videos

Videos, an increasingly popular form of health education, are made and replaced more rapidly than books. Therefore, it makes sense to think of the titles that follow as examples of the kinds of materials available and to check the current catalogues of the organizations that produce or market them.

Videos distributed by the American Diabetes Association

Beyond Injection: Living with An Insulin Pump
The Black Experience
Diabetes: A Positive Approach
Diabetes & Exercise Video
Diabetes and You
Diabetes In Your School or Child Care Center
Diabetes Update—Glucose Toxicity: The Need for 24-Hour Control
Diabetes: What You Need to Know
The Diabetic Foot
Emergency Medical Training
Introduction to the Exchange System
Label Reading and Shopping
Living Well with Diabetes
On Top of My Game: Living with Diabetes
Physicians' Guide to Type I Diabetes
Understanding Diabetes – a User's Guide to Novolin
Understanding Diabetes and Living a Healthy Life

Videos distributed by the Joslin Diabetes Center

Armchair Fitness: Aerobics
Know Your Diabetes, Know Yourself
Living with Diabetes: A Winning Formula

American Association of Diabetes Educators Video Series

Diabetes and Exercise: In Training
Diabetes and Nutrition: Eating for Health
Introduction to Diabetes: The Game Plan

Other Sources

Novo Nordisk Diabetes Care Videos
Time/Life Medical

Periodicals

Journals and Newsletters Published by the American Diabetes Association

Clinical Diabetes (a newsletter for primary-care physicians)

Diabetes (a scholarly journal focusing on biomedical research)

The Diabetes Advisor (current medical developments for professionals and patients)

Diabetes Care (a journal on clinical-care issues addressed to health professionals but accessible to the interested lay reader)

Diabetes Forecast (a very readable magazine for people with diabetes and their families – includes *Kids' Corner*)

Diabetes Reviews (literature reviews for professionals on scientific and clinical questions)

Diabetes Spectrum: From Research to Practice (summarizes research findings and applies them to clinical practice)

Journals and Newsletters Published by Other Organizations

Countdown (Juvenile Diabetes Foundation International: news updates for parents and professionals)

Diabetes Educator (American Association of Diabetes Educators: information for health professionals with emphasis on patient education and counseling)

Diabetes Self-Management (R.A. Rapaport Publishing, Inc.: practical how-to information in an upbeat style for people with diabetes)

N.D.I.C. Newsletter (National Diabetes Information Clearinghouse: the latest developments and trends)

Organizations Providing Support in Coping with Various Aspects of Diabetes

Some of the organizations listed here have web sites listed previously under the heading "On the World Wide Web."

ABLEDATA
8455 Colesville Rd., Suite 935
Silver Spring, MD 20910-3319
(800) 227-0216
(Information clearinghouse for assistive technology and rehabilitation equipment)

Agency for Health Care Policy and Research (AHCPR)
Medical Treatment Effectiveness Program
Division of Information and Publications
2101 East Jefferson Avenue
Rockville, MD 20852
(301) 227-8364

American Association of Diabetes Educators
444 N. Michigan Avenue, Suite 1240
Chicago, IL 60611-3901
(312) 644-2233
(800) 338-3633
(Upon written request, this organization will provide information
about diabetes education in your area.)

American Association of Sex Educators, Counselors, and
Therapists
P.O. Box 238
Mt. Vernon, IA 52314-0238
(319) 895-8407
(Will provide recommendations for counselors in your vicinity)

American Dental Association
Bureau of Dental Health Education
211 East Chicago Avenue
Chicago, IL 60611
(312) 440-2500
(Supplies information about dental care and hygiene)

American Diabetes Association
1660 Duke St.
Alexandria, VA 22314
(703) 549-1500
(800) 232-3472
(Local affiliates can be contacted by calling 1-800-DIABETES.)

American Dietetic Association
216 West Jackson Blvd., Suite 800
Chicago, IL 60606
(312) 899-0040
(800) 366-1655
(A professional organization that can help find a local nutritionist)

American Foundation for the Blind
11 Penn Plaza, Suite 300
New York, NY 10001
(212) 502-7600
(212) 947-1060
(800) 232-5463

American Heart Association
7272 Greenville Avenue
Dallas, TX 75231
(800) 242-8721

American Kidney Fund
6110 Executive Boulevard, Suite 1010
Rockville, MD 20852-3915
(301) 881-3052
(800) 638-8299

American Podiatric Medical Association
9312 Old Georgetown Road
Bethesda, MD 20814-1698
(301) 571-9200

American Printing House for the Blind
P.O. Box 6085
Louisville, Ky 40206-0085
(502) 895-2405
(800) 223-1839
(Supplies large-print books, cassettes, and educational aids)

American Psychiatric Association
1400 K Street, N.W.
Washington, DC 20005-2492
(202) 682-6000

Americans With Disabilities Act Information
(800) ADA-WORK

Americans With Disabilities Act Technical Assistance Centers
U.S. Department of Justice
(800) 949-4232
(Ten regional centers offering information and guidance on the
Americans With Disabilities Act)

Association for the Education and Rehabilitation of the Blind and
Visually Impaired
206 N. Washington St., Suite 320
Alexandria, VA 22314
(703) 823-9690

Garfield G. Duncan Research Foundation, Inc.
Diabetes Information Center
829 Spruce Street, Suite 302
Philadelphia, PA 19107-5752
(215) 829-3426

Equal Employment Opportunity Commission
1801 L St., N.W.
Washington, DC 20507
(800) 669-4000

Family Voices
P.O. Box 769
Algodones, NM 87001
(505) 867-2368
(Provides information, referrals, and advocacy to improve health
care for children with disabilities)

Federation for Children with Special Needs
95 Berkeley St., Suite 104
Boston, MA 02116
(617) 482-2915
(800) 331-0688 (MA only)
(An information and referral agency, including directories of local support services, for parents of children with special health care needs)

Health Insurance Association of America (HIAA)
555 13th St., N.W., Suite 600 East
Washington, DC 20004
(202) 824-1600
(Provides free booklets such as *The Consumer's Guide to Health Insurance, The Consumer's Guide to Long-Term Care Insurance, The Consumer's Guide to Medicare Supplement Insurance*, and *The Consumer's Guide to Disability Supplement Insurance*)

International Diabetic Athletes Association
1647 W. Bethany Home Rd., #B
Phoenix, AZ 85015
(602) 433-2113
(800) 898-IDAA

Job Accommodation Network
President's Committee on Employment of People with Disabilities
918 Chestnut Ridge Rd., Suite 1
Morgantown, WV 26505
(800) 526-7234
(Offers information and resources for individuals and employers on disability rights, employability, and job accommodation)

Joslin Diabetes Center
One Joslin Place
Boston, MA 02215
(617) 732-2400

Juvenile Diabetes Foundation International
120 Wall Street, 19th Floor
New York, NY 10005-3904
(212) 785-9500
(800) 223-1138
(Check for local community chapters)

Medic Alert Foundation International
2323 Colorado Ave.
Turlock, CA 95382
(800) 432-5378
(800) 344-3226
(Manufactures medical identification tags and bracelets)

National Association for the Visually Handicapped (NAVH)
22 West 21st Street
New York, NY 10010
(212) 889-3141

National Association for the Visually Handicapped (NAVH)
3201 Balboa Street
San Francisco, CA 94121
(415) 221-3201
(Supplies vision care information, referrals, and support services;
provides visual aids, large-print publications, and information on
commercial printers)

National Center for Chronic Disease Prevention and Health
Promotion
Centers for Disease Control (CDC)
1600 Clifton Road, N.E.
The Rodes Building, MS K-13
Atlanta, GA 30333
(404) 639-3311

National Diabetes Information Clearinghouse
Box NDIC
1 Information Way
Bethesda, MD 20892
(301) 654-3327
(Upon request, will supply a bibliography of all literature on diabetes)

National Eye Health Education Program
National Eye Institute, National Institutes of Health
Box 20/20
Bethesda, MD 20892
(301) 496-5248

National Federation of the Blind
1800 Johnson Street
Baltimore, MD 21230-4998
(410) 659-9314
(A membership organization, performs advocacy work; provides information as well as aids for blind and visually impaired persons)

National Institutes of Health
U.S. Dept. of Health and Human Services
9000 Rockville Pike
Bethesda, MD 20892-0002
(301) 496-4000

National Institute of Mental Health
Public Inquiries Office
17C17 Parklawn Building
5600 Fishers Lane
Rockville, MD 20857-0001
(301) 443-3175
(Funds research and awards grants, with particular interest in research on the emotional aspects of diabetes)

National Kidney Foundation
30 E. 33rd St.
New York, NY 10016
(212) 889-2210
(800) 622-9010

National Library Service for the Blind and Physically Handicapped
U.S. Library of Congress
1291 Taylor Street, N.W.
Washington, DC 20542-4960
(202) 707-5100

National Rehabilitation Information Center (NARIC)
8455 Colesville Rd., Suite 935
Silver Spring, MD 20910-3319
(301) 588-9284
(800) 346-2742
(Maintains databases on disability and rehabilitation)

Recordings for the Blind and Dyslexic
20 Roszel Road
Princeton, NJ 08540
(609) 452-0606
(800) 221-4792 (business hours)

U.S. Dept. of Health and Human Services
200 Independence Avenue, S.W.
Washington, DC 20201
(202) 619-0257

U.S. Government Technical Information Services Branch
(404) 488-5080
(Supplies information on surveillance and prevention of diabetes
for health-care professionals and people with diabetes)

Vision Foundation, Inc.
818 Mount Auburn Street
Watertown, MA 02472-1567
(617) 926-4232
(MA only) (800) 852-3029

Index

media coverage of diabetes, 8
   See also public awareness of
      diabetes
medical conditions due to diabetes, 8
   See also amputations; blind-
      ness; coma; complica-
      tions; deaths; heart
      disease; kidney disease;
      nerve disease; sexual
      dysfunction; vision
      impairment
medications for diabetes, 42
   prescription problems, 129–31
   unnecessary (in type 2), 6
   See also insulin; oral medica-
      tions
metformin (biguanides), 37, 228
misconceptions about diabetes,
   9, 25–28

nasal spray devices, 225
Native Americans and diabetes,
   8
needles. *See* insulin injections
nephropathy. *See* kidney disease
nerve disease, 41, 105, 248
neuropathy. *See* nerve disease
non-insulin-dependent diabetes, 34
noninvasive testing, 226
nurses as caregivers, 139–40,
   143–44
nutrition. *See* diet and nutrition

obesity, 8, 33, 37, 59
   compulsive eating, 77–80
   emotions and, 64
   See also weight control

online resources, 236–37,
   291–93
openness and secrecy, 84–90
oral medications, 37, 248
   changes in, 228
   type 2 and, 112–13
overcompensation, 61
   with children, 181–83
overprotectiveness, 150–51, 162,
   179–82

pancreas, 33, 224, 248
   beta cell transplants, 224–25
patient-doctor relations. *See* doc-
      tor-patient relations
parents of diabetic children,
   169–70
   anxiety, 172–73
   case studies, 86–88, 240
      See also Chapter 8
   conflict points, 171–72
   diet of the family, 187–8
   emotional distancing, 55
   emotional problems, 64
   guilt and, 50, 173–77
   heredity, 173–74
   independence vs. dependence,
      179, 182–83
   insulin injection and, 85
   insulin issues, 171, 182–83
   issues for, 179–85
   limit testing, 183–85
   needs of, 185–87
   overcompensation, 181–83
   overprotectiveness, 179–81
   travel and recreation issues,
      216–18
peripheral vascular disease, 40

About the Authors

Jerry Edelwich, L.C.S.W., is Director of the New England Association of Reality Therapy and coordinator of employee assistance programs at Anthem Blue Cross/Blue Shield of Connecticut. He teaches, consults, and conducts workshops throughout the world on living with diabetes as well as on individual and group counseling skills, drug and alcohol rehabilitation, sexual issues in professional relationships, and staff burnout. He is coauthor (with Archie Brodsky) of *Burnout: Stages of Disillusionment in the Helping Professions; Sexual Dilemmas for the Helping Professional;* and *Group Counseling for the Resistant Client.*

Archie Brodsky is senior research associate in the Program in Psychiatry and the Law, Harvard Medical School at Massachusetts Mental Health Center, where he has served as chair of the Human Rights Committee. In addition to his books with Jerry Edelwich, he is coauthor of *Love and Addiction; The Truth About Addiction and Recovery; Medical Choices, Medical Chances;* and numerous other books and journal articles in psychology and medicine.

For information concerning workshops for professionals or lay persons on the emotional and practical aspects of diabetes, please contact:

Jerry Edelwich, L.C.S.W.
234 South Main Street, Suite 402
Middletown, CT 06457
(860) 347-3836 (phone/FAX)
e-mail: NEART @aol.com

develop a Concrete image in a
persons mind can do more
to galvanize change and
motivate better choices
than all the statistics the
mind can build   Amen

"septemistic option suicide"

by making harmful choices

gradually unwittingly
undramatically damages
our choices here & now
even people who appear to be
among the worlds most educated

here are their reasons